The Medical Manager

The Medical Manager

A practical guide for clinicians

Anthony E Young

Guy's and St Thomas' Hospital Trust, St Thomas' Hospital, London, UK

40643

© BMJ Books 1999
BMJ Books is an imprint of the BMJ Publishing Group

First published in 1999
by BMJ Books, BMA House, Tavistock Square,
London WC1H 9JR

British Library Cataloguing in Publication Data

A catalogue record for this book is available from the
British Library

ISBN 0-7279-1376-X

Typeset, printed and bound in Great Britain by
Latimer Trend & Company Ltd, Plymouth

Contents

Preface

We live our lives forwards, we explain them backwards. This book, in part, is the explaining backwards of eight years spent in medical management; the first four as Director of Surgical Services, the second four as a Medical Director of Guy's & St Thomas' Hospital Trust. In explaining backwards and advising forwards one's views are bound to be coloured by a set of beliefs, and I admit at the outset a belief in the NHS as a public service; in the context of an under-funded, poorly directed service it is very effective (as distinct from efficient). However, the NHS has faults for which everyone in it, not just politicians, is partly responsible. Doctors have traditionally played a role in guiding the service in the right direction and helping it to withstand the short-term ideological obsessions of politicians and attempts to short-change the NHS and those that it serves. Their primacy in this managerial role is no longer as clear as it was, and they need to renew their belief in that role and their skills at achieving it. Hence this book is written for sceptics who do not regard management by clinicians as appropriate, for doctors in training and, lastly, for those who are freshly into clinical management posts and looking for some "street knowledge".

I hope this book will help those who wish to help guide the service by involving themselves in the day-to-day management of it. The text may seem somewhat didactic but that is its purpose for my intention was to make this a practical guide. Much of what I have written I did not know when I first became a medical manager (I wish I had), and most of what I have written has been learned from experience or I have found that experience has fitted with current theory. Where experience has been at variance with what is in the books I have said so. In those disagreements I have not claimed to be the little boy commenting on the emperor's clothes, I have merely noted that the clothes are nowhere near as grand as they are claimed. The little boy of the story was no doubt taken home and soundly spanked, and I expect some of what I have to say will be seen by acolytes of the management revolution as either reprehensible ignorance or an inability to comprehend the true path to the glorious future. That would be sad, as some of the preoccupations of managerialism stand to destroy as much good as they may create.

This is essentially a single-author book so I have, perhaps, been lopsided in my stress on certain subjects which have concerned me to the neglect of others which have been less interesting or less problematical. Nevertheless, I hope I have covered the ground across which the medical manager exercises his or her responsibilities. In doing so I have deliberately dwelt on those topics which affect the medical manager in his or her proper role as an intermediary between medicine and management. Conversely I have minimised reference to purely managerial issues such as personnel, finance and contracting which are dealt with at length in other books on clinical management. The territory is necessarily viewed predominantly from an acute hospital perspective, but surveys of medical managers' work shows homogeneous activities, problems and aspirations across all types of hospital and health authority.

Note on terminology: I have used the term "medical management" at its most general, meaning any form of management with which doctors may become involved. I have used the term "clinical management" to cover the more specific activity of a clinician managing a clinical directorate or team.

Note for doctors in training

This is not a textbook of management practice, but you do not need such a textbook any more than a non-clinical manager needs a textbook of medicine. This book is intended to give you a feel for what medical management is about and also contains practical tips for those about to become actively involved. As a trainee looking at the business of management from the outside you may have been confused by the competing passions of the objectors on one side and the management acolytes on the other. It does not matter with which side your natural sympathies lie because the economic and managerial aspects of medical practice are inescapable, so you will need to have a feel for the issues. Very few doctors in the future Health Service will find that they can ignore the pressure to become involved in practical managerial tasks and most senior trainees know that the chief executive and medical director of the trust in which they are seeking a consultant job will probably be on the advisory appointments committee! (or their representatives will). These managers will not unreasonably expect a positive as well as an informed attitude to management issues; indeed some appointment processes now set candidates a task that involves a mock business planning exercise. May I suggest, therefore, that if you are skimming this book you flit through Chapter 1 then skip to Chapter 3, looking at Sections 3.5 Managing a budget, 3.6 Business planning and 3.7 Managing for quality, for the important general topics. Section 4.3 in Chapter 4 deals with managing conflict, Section 4.6 is about difficult colleagues, and the whole of Chapter 6 covers the sort of problem areas in which you might be expected to take a view. Lastly Chapter 5 about the NHS as an institution has some background information which may help you to structure your views of the NHS in the general context of a public service. I hope that at the end of all that you will have enough of a feel for the issues to be able to make your own informed judgments.

Acknowledgments

I would never have thought to write this book if it were not for the stimulating good fellowship of colleagues at St Thomas' and at Guy's, principally Tim Matthews, John Pelly, Wilma McPherson, Tim Higginson and Matt Tee, the other clinicians in management, also John Parkes, Rosemary Burch and Elizabeth Browse, and the hordes of sceptical doctors and nurses outside management whose apposite questioning usually kept our feet on the ground. I am particularly grateful to Nicol Thin for his section on the management of health service research, to Brian Ayers for elucidating the new GMC professional performance procedures and to John Pelly for overseeing the sections on finance. Also to Jenny Simpson, Chief Executive of the British Association of Medical Managers (BAMM) who has been an inspirational force for many whose enthusiasm for the hard graft of management has begun to flag. I am grateful to Marion Gill and Heather Nicholls for their secretarial support and to the publishing skills of those at BMJ Books. Lastly, and above all others, to my wife who in difficult times never wavered in her support and without whose encouragement this book would never have been completed.

AEY
London, September 1998

Introduction

Many clinicians hold a sceptical or even frankly negative view of medical management, yet many will wittingly or unwittingly be swept into medical management posts or wish to find out more. Unfortunately, if they look for guidance they may find themselves immediately uncomfortable with the unquestioning faith in managerialism and medical management expressed in most books on the subject. The introductory chapter to one such book is entitled "On the Road to Damascus".[1]

Many doctors harbour a perception that for a clinician to be a manager is to desert his true calling, that clinical management is a disreputable even degrading job, and that the motives for doing it are at best incomprehensible and at worst an exercise in self aggrandisement. I overstate the case, but not by as much as you might think. The reader of books and articles about medical management will find no inkling of the suspicion and anxiety that colours so many clinicians' views; such publications are hallmarked with a halcyon image of a man in a grey suit and a man in a white coat arm in arm with the woman with big shoulder pads striding purposefully into the roseate dawn of the sweetly managed health service. The books contain a wealth of information to help this happy trio carry out their jobs ever better, but almost never do they address the gut feelings of disquiet and frustration felt by most clinicians. These books are predicated on the assumption that the faults in the Health Service are due to archaic attitudes and practices within the service and could be solved if only every clinician could be taught to "understand management". By contrast, I hope that this book will address those clinicians' anxieties and the causes for them. I have not replicated the tone of other books on management nor covered the field in the same way. I have dwelt somewhat on the areas most clinicians find difficult, irritating or particularly opaque, and have avoided other purely technical areas where all that would be needed is a reference book. Nevertheless, you should not expect this book to feed all your

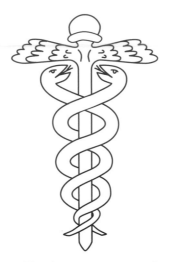

Figure 1.1   The Caduceus. The wings represent transcendence, diligence and activity. The Wand represents power, the axis mundi down which messages travel between heaven and earth. The double serpents represent the dualist opposites, healing versus poison, illness versus health. They also represent Mediation between the upper and lower realms, Good and Evil. Altogether the perfect symbol of office for the medical manager, interlocutor and healer.

antimanagerial prejudices or debunk the need for doctors in management. The thesis of this book is simple: firstly doctors have the aptitude and the knowledge to enable them to be managers or to integrate with managers; secondly they have an obligation to do so as one of the means towards fulfilling their primary task—the proper care of patients, and lastly they can do so without selling their souls to their imaginary devil. In accepting the need to be involved with or as managers they should nevertheless console themselves with the fact that although much is wrong with the Health Service, much is also wrong with some of the remedies and the way they are administered. Doctors need to help get it right. The interwoven serpents of the physician's symbol, the caduceus, do after all symbolise healing through the balancing of opposing forces (Figure 1.1).[2]

> We need not fall victim to the liberal fallacy of assuming that because we can perceive a problem we are, *de facto*, not part of the problem.
>
> DAVID MAMET on "Decay"[3]

References

1 Grime P. In: Lees P, ed. *Navigating the NHS*. Abingdon: Radcliffe Medical Press, 1996.
2 Cooper JC. *Encyclopedia of Traditional Symbols*. London: Thames and Hudson, 1978.
3 Mamet D. Decay: some thoughts for action. In: *A Whore's Profession*. London: Faber and Faber, 1992, pp. 186–92.

1 Doctors as Managers

1.1 Management and the profession of medicine

To understand why so many clinicians are dissatisfied and why they focus so much of this dissatisfaction on to managers and the process of management, one needs to look back to see what has been happening over the past 15 years. "Too many managers" is seen simplistically as the problem, when analysis shows it is the *managerialism* of which they are merely a symptom that is the true cause of the unhappiness. The core of that managerialism is the presumption that the failings of the Health Service are a result of attitudes and processes that are fundamentally flawed and could be solved by the imposition of a new order by managers. This "new order", this managerialism, is a mix of an obsession with control, accountability and measurement overlaid onto a hotch potch of different business management theories imported into the public sector, historically late and frequently inappropriately. For clinicians as for other professionals the real damage is done by the consequential lack of professional autonomy which denies their professionalism and goes cheek by jowl with a progressive loss of power. It is not easy to separate the loss of *professionalism* from the loss of *power*, but any would-be manager needs to understand clinicians' views about this erosion of status professionally and within the organisation. He also needs to understand how the new finance- and efficiency-based managerialism can damage the public service values of the people it affects, leading to a deterioration in morale and performance which overshadows the benefits that are supposed to accrue. Private sector management theory is not transportable to public services without major modification.[1]

A crude summary of Luke's thesis of the three dimensions of power[2] identifies them as:

● Controlling the agenda.
● Controlling expectations.
● Controlling the players.

1

The medical profession's dominance in each of these areas shrinks daily. I know that most managers would say that doctors still have an inappropriately powerful stranglehold on the delivery of health care and find it difficult to understand clinicians' anxieties. They may not perceive how the culture of managerialism is insidiously taking over territory previously solely within the clinician's demesne and even in quite small details denying his power to judge what process of care is best for patients. This is not a phenomenon solely experienced by doctors but is simply an expression of a wider trend in society as the power, status and privileges of the professions are eroded. Within the Health Service some of the territorial incursions are inadvertent, such as changes to the processes of appointment and rotation of junior staff and the way beds are now managed. These changes with many others can mean that the clinician no longer feels he has an accountable staff and a defined physical territory and is increasingly uncertain about his prerogatives, even when face to face with a patient. It all contributes to the demoralisation that can lead to poor performance at one end of the scale or bolshie confrontationalism at the other. At the very least it feeds the antimanagerial culture prevalent among clinicians—70% of doctors are reported as antipathetic to managers. In exploring this further the cherished notion of a clinician's professionalism is itself worth exploring.

1.1.1 Professionalism and its erosion

We need to understand what we mean when as doctors we describe ourselves as *professionals*. At its simplest we imply an exclusive, collegiate grouping defining and administering a set of skills. It is a social as much as a technical phenomenon, but a profession derives its power from those skills, unlike the bureaucrat who derives power primarily from his position. Doctors tend to admit only one view of their professional ethos, the humanistic, caring view, and indeed it is important that they do so for there are other opinions which identify our professionalism as simply an exercise in self interest or just as an unhelpful social phenomenon. But more of this later; first to flesh out the traditional view, the average doctor's self image.

The doctors' view of professionalism

> NHS doctors do not accept that they are working "under" anyone outside the profession, only within the managerial framework of a public service and the professional constraints laid on them by the General Medical Council; they work for patients.
>
> (LEE–POTTER[3])

Within the ambit of one's professionalism as a clinician one might properly claim to know about disease and its treatment and about what patients need and want; but one quite reasonably might also claim to know how best to define and deliver the services which affect those patients and their illnesses. Also one could claim some primacy in knowing how best to educate and choose one's successors. The margins of all these areas are being nibbled away. There is a hazier area concerning professionalism which is to do with personal conduct and the emotional and physical commitment that a doctor makes to patients. By claiming with nurses sole occupancy of this high ground some doctors are encouraged to believe that there is an automatic rightness in their judgment which cannot be questioned by others; an inheritance of moral authority somewhat akin to Roman Catholic priestship. It is this sense of responsibility in certain areas of medicine that motivates clinicians. Training, education, experience and character are perceived as the mainsprings of proper care for patients, as validating leadership of the team and giving the right to define the shape of the future of medicine. With a few notable exceptions doctors tend to view this congruent set of skills, activities and privileges as uniquely theirs. These are indeed the components of their professionalism. Autonomy is a crucial element in this because the relationship between a patient or a client and a professional is characterised by the patient's minimal or absent knowledge about her problems and her need to enter into a dependent relationship with the doctor. In order to provide an environment in which this trust is not exploited the professional must be able to act free from outside interference and he must also be free to regulate his profession to protect it from charlatans and the incompetent. Lastly where there is a team dealing with clinical matters he asserts a right to be the leader of that team.

Managers' professionalism

Non-medical managers also perceive themselves as professionals but, by contrast, they see themselves as having universal skills

3

in organisation, finance, planning, people, education. Not unreasonably, they are trained to believe that these skills are portable and that most managers are totipotent, as applicable in a hospital as in a bank or a business. They do not demand autonomy; indeed, they can only exist of part of a hierarchical system of interdependent teams.

When the managers' area of influence overlaps with that of doctors there is bound to be trouble. From the clinician's point of view the overlap was not originally overlap but simply juxta-position, which was when *managers* were *administrators*—passive implementers of a static set of operational arrangements and clearly lower in the pecking order than doctors. But managers do not want to be administrators they want to be managers. They hate the term administrator and indeed to call a manager an administrator is the quickest and most predictable way to annoy. Real managers want to make things happen differently. They live by change and for change. If nothing changes they do indeed simply become administrators (in effect they usually just leave). Change is the engine, the tonic, the aphrodisiac and as we are living in an era of continuous change in medicine, the manager quickly becomes a major player on a level with the clinician. Change is not perceived by the clinician as central to his life in medicine. Change is not a feature of the core activity; cancers are still cut out, diabetes is still treated with insulin, fractures plastered and leaky valves replaced.

When managerialism first began to intrude into clinical practice it was into those areas at the edge of the medical empire where the clinician's hold is less confident—the organisation of care delivery, priority setting, education, finance. Most recently the incursions have become bolder and will become more so; for example, a proposal of the 1998 white paper that managers should become directly responsible for service quality will *de facto* involve them in the details of clinical practice. What troubles doctors is not so much the fact of change as the details of change and the reality that change is predominantly commissioned and led at all levels by non-doctors and, furthermore, that those non-doctors are increasingly questioning how the doctor does things.

If you wish to assess the effect this is having on doctors simply look around you, read the non-clinical parts of the journals, the letters columns, talk to doctors and managers and ask how many clinicians have planned early retirement. A BMA survey of 800 doctors in April 1996 found that seven out of ten suffered from

4

work-related stress and 88% considered they were more stressed than they had been 5 years earlier. Of those reporting work-related stress more than 25% had increased their alcohol intake to help them cope and one in five had contemplated suicide.[4] Another study found that whereas increasing seniority was previously associated with less stress that now seems to be reversed, higher stress levels being reported in consultants than house officers.[5] A separate and more scientific assessment by Ramirez also reported high stress levels and identified the top three causes of stress as work overload, feeling poorly managed and resourced and, lastly, the impact of managerial responsibilities. The authors confirmed that "the transfer of various responsibilities from clinicians to managers may undermine professional morale".[6] Another study has shown that two-thirds of general practice principals had considered leaving general practice, the commonest reason being "increasing bureaucracy/government interference".[7] And do not think it is just the old fogies too sclerotic to accept healthy change. Isobel Allen of the Policies Studies Institute studied the "core values" of doctors under forty ("Committed but Critical"). Her conclusion was that young doctors are developing a widespread sense of isolation and alienation caused chiefly by the managerial culture within the NHS:

> These young doctors want their professional competence and clinical judgment to be respected.

Other research by the Policy Studies Institute has shown a worrying acceleration in the number of young doctors who regret their decision to study medicine, a rise from 26% of male graduates in 1976 to 58% of 1986 graduates and, appallingly, a rise from 30% for 1976 female graduates to 76% for the 1986 cohort.[8] Many stresses account for this but many are in the areas encompassed by managerialism and deprofessionalisation. A survey of psychiatrists who elected to retire early gave their reasons as "increasing bureaucracy, government policies, the internal market and interference by managers".[9]

The focal point of the clinician's professionalism is an assumed right of pre-eminence in defining what is the correct and incorrect treatment for illnesses, and all her powers flow from that. However even at this centre point of medical professionalism the clinician's primacy is being challenged by managers empowered by evidence-based medicine, emboldened by holding the budget or the power to define a contract. Once that core area in clinical professionalism

5

is invaded by others the clinician potentially becomes a mere technologist, a creature of protocols and service specifications. The continued sniping by the media and their ill-informed promotion of alternative medicine adds to the overall feeling of a profession under threat. Crucially there is also a self-destructive effect from the widespread cynicism that clinicians have in their interpretation of most management-driven reforms. Normally announced as improvements in quality or quantity of service for patients, clinicians usually perceive these simply as concealed attempts at cost savings. All this sounds very unhappy, very unsatisfactory and clearly needs to be addressed. Indeed this is the true crisis in the Health Service. Deprofessionalisation is the germ that has infected the system and has the power to devitalise it progressively over the next few years. We are already seeing it in the changed attitudes of younger trainees. This would not itself be a fatal infection but would certainly weaken the ability to fight the effects of under-funding and continued change. The service, of course, would not collapse but the quality of care may deteriorate and the quantity needed will be delivered only grudgingly. What are we to do then?

1.1.2 Redefining professionalism

Clinicians (doctors who touch patients) must redefine their professionalism and incorporate in the new definition a concept of understanding citizenship as well as individualism. Additionally they will need to embrace the management of change and be able to manage that change effectively and constructively. They will need to learn to work humbly in teams and accept that others besides doctors have valid views about how best to provide medical care. They will need to share with non-clinical managers those marginal areas mentioned earlier and to regard the contributions of those managers as potentially constructive rather than solely destructive. To do so they are going to have to learn to be effective in those areas themselves, and most are going to have to become managers in one form or another while still being doctors. The paradox and the irony of this is that redemption from their anxieties about managers lies in becoming one. On the other side of the divide the government, health authorities, public health doctors and non-clinical managers are going to have to learn the difference between a doctor and a manager and are going to have to modulate their enthusiasm for change for the sake of change. If doctors are

6

not faced by successive waves of futile change and unimplementable dictats or cost controls dressed up as quality improvement, they may be able to adjust to the new environment, redefine their professionalism and regain their morale; possibly even their primacy in the system. It is a lesson of history as well as of biology that success comes only through adaptation.

Other interpretations of medical professionalism

In the 1960s and 1970s the much quoted "Medical nemesis" by Ivan Illich[10] was centred on the claim that the profession and science of medicine far from improving the health of society was in fact superfluous. That view is no longer fashionable nor scientifically tenable, but clinicians should be aware of two other interpretations of medical professionalism which social scientists like to air.

The first might be called the "Monopolistic Control" view.

> It is argued that professionals...actually act in pursuit of self interest rather than client/patient interest. Thus the characteristics of professionalism such as autonomy and self regulation help to produce a situation in which managerial control and supervision can be evaded, and in which the practice of specific skills can be retained as a monopoly within the profession, helping keep earnings higher, and career prospects better than would otherwise have been the case.[11]

This fits well with the simplistic tenet of "Rational Choice theory", which was fashionable with social scientists in the 1980s—all rational choices are informed only by "knavish" self interest and that financial gain is at its heart. This in turn harmonises with the "Thatcherite" tenets of individualism and belief in the pervasive powers of "the market". Fortunately for those who believe altruism is alive and well subsequent "research" has cast doubt on this most cynical of theories.

The second might be termed a "Neo-Marxist" view and identifies the habits of medical professionalism as secondary to social conditioning. Doctors are selected mainly from middle class backgrounds and are educated within a social elite, they thus take on traditional authority values and continue to reinforce them throughout their careers.[12] Nurses have accepted and mimicked this hierarchical arrangement and patients are conditioned socially to accept it uncritically as an advantageous norm. Furthermore,

7

the ills of society are "medicalised" such that they become attributes of individuals, not of society as a whole. The hospital becomes symbolic of this as well as of the social power of the medical and nursing professions.[13] Lastly the political embarrassment of diseases, whether caused by the social structure of the state or unresolved because of rationing or inequitable access, is concealed and mollified by an acquiescent medical profession acting as an agent of the state.[14]

You should know about these alternative and often deeply cynical views of your behaviour, if only because you may find them used to rationalise power struggles or salve the consciences of those who, for honourable or dishonourable motives, may wish to diminish the status of the medical profession. You might also note a not infrequent whiff of class war sentiment in some of what is written about the management of health care; an unadmitted, unconstructive undercurrent.

1.2 Doctors and managers—two tribes?

It has been said that "management is an activity, not a social group", but managers within the Health Service are an identifiable separate group of people. You are a doctor, you will probably remain a doctor, yet in some ways you will need to become a manager, a different profession with different skills addressing a different type of problem using different styles and methods for dealing with them. To some extent you will be play acting for as long as you are managing. The professional manager will know this and your relationship with him may be a fruitful journey of mutual support and education, or it may be an unhappy paranoid relationship that you both are relieved, in due course, to escape from. In my experience several issues can sour the relationship. Perhaps the most common is where the newly appointed clinical director thinks he can breeze into management and be totipotent and effective from the first day; hiring and firing, spending and cutting. This is rarely so. Secondly, the new clinical director may constantly behave as if he is not really part of the management team, feeling able to swing in and out, support or resist initiatives as the mood or expediency takes him. These habits are likely to irritate the less well paid but just as hard working and professional manager. Conversely the management tribe may upset the doctor in management by expecting him to "come across", leaving behind all his clinician's reflexes and sensitivities. There is no reason why a clinician should not become a perfectly good manager without the need for total cultural assimilation. The clinician—manager relationship need not be a *folie a deux* in which both can only coexist because they support each others' delusions. Clinicians need to learn the language of management and to work with managers but not to parody them. Managers and doctors do after all largely share the same objectives and perhaps also the same character attributes which have been identified for doctors by John Butterfield:

(1) courage
(2) intelligence
(3) wisdom
(4) style

to which I would add

(5) optimism

For all this doctors and managers remain two separate tribes and it does not help to demand that they are the same. The following lists caricature some of the differences.

Doctors	**Managers**
Moral absolutists	Moral relativists
Deal in specifics	Deal in the general
Autonomous decision taker	Group decision taker
Conservative, suspicious of change	Thrive on change
Scientific	Non-scientific
Long stay in post	Short stay in post

1.2.1 Intellectual equivalence?

The process of medical decision taking is relatively straightforward. There is one patient at a time to consider using a body of evidence obtained from examining and investigating the patient. That evidence has to be weighed and sifted according to the doctor's knowledge and experience and a management (note the word!) decision made by the doctor using all her experience and knowledge finally modulated by a humanitarian view of this particular patient's needs. Then on to the next patient. Medicine's problems come in neat packages called patients and they can be dealt with quite

9

quickly and one at a time. It is a little difficult, therefore, to understand why clinicians can be so arrogantly dismissive of the intellectual skills of other forms of management. Many of the problems that managers grapple with are more complex, more difficult to analyse, less easily soluble by formula and carry the added difficulty that implementation of the management plan requires more stamina and greater use of interpersonal skills than is ever called upon in the clinical context. None of this need matter to the clinician turned manager. However, it is likely to depress or anger him on discovering that colleagues have employed the same squiffy quality judgments to deny the validity of managerial decisions he has taken, or to exclude him from inclusion in a merit awards nominations list!

1.2.2 Moral relativism

This high-sounding title identifies a crucial difference between managers and clinicians, an inherent difference which cannot be made to go away by debate. The difference is a factor in the discomfort many clinicians feel about being in managerial posts. At its simplest the clinician believes she is the servant of a set of moral absolutes concerning the care of patients. The clinician maintains an idealised view of her relationship with the patient, a sort of heroic one-to-one relationship unsullied by commerce, error or the vagaries of human communication. For example, the clinician believes that every patient is entitled to every jot of treatment that might be available, that the treatment should be available promptly and that the stay in hospital should be governed by the true social, personal and medical needs of the patient. There are no such absolutes for the relativist manager, nor can there be. The relativist manager must work within limited resources and cut his cloth appropriately, he must work in a landscape of continuous change and uncertainty. Clinicians increasingly accept the reality of this situation but it does not mean that they like it, and they believe that to espouse it formally by taking up a management post will run counter to their professional commitment to provide the best available care for all patients. They also identify another argument beyond the simple adherence to a finite budget, and they are anxious that as managers they may be put in a position where they must implement polices that are the product not of economics but of political ideology or whim which may work against a patient's true needs. One can share managers' irritation at the overstatement of the moral case that some doctors make. There are too many doctors who seem to be happy to spend their time picnicking on the moral high ground, simply chucking stones at those toiling on the lower slopes trying to raise the staple crop. Nevertheless, all need to admit that there is a real and irreconcilable difference of emphasis . . . which is actually useful.

Nor should doctors complain at the appearance on the scene of so many managers. When Sir Roy Griffiths was collecting evidence for his report on NHS management,[15] doctors were not slow to point out how undermanaged as well as ineptly managed the NHS was. They observed that there seemed to be few effective mechanisms for getting things done. This indeed was the thrust of Griffiths' final report. In his oft-quoted summary of the situation Roy Griffiths said "if Florence Nightingale were carrying her lamp through the corridors of the NHS today she would almost certainly be searching for the people in charge". That report ended a period of formal consensus management in the NHS and heralded the 18 000 rise in the number of NHS managers between 1989 and 1994 and an increase in the managerial pay bill over the same period from £158.8 m. to £723.3 m. The actual total health authority and NHS trust management costs for 1995/6 in England were £1773 million.[16] "Nowadays you can't shine your lamp into any part of the organisation without revealing a crowd of people who are supposed to be in charge".[17] It's worth noting though that Griffiths foresaw the need for doctors in managerial posts and holding and being specifically responsible for budgets.

Lastly one should be insightful and frank about the negative attitudes that many clinicians have to change or novelty and how they have let go of the helm during the difficult last ten years of the Health Service, allowing the initiative to be shaped by politicians, academic social scientists, economists and managers. We must not be surprised at this, nor prepared to tolerate it. Jeremy Lee-Potter, erstwhile Chairman of the BMA wrote:[18]

> The window dressing from ministers about involving doctors in management is largely tinsel. Lions led by donkeys have a habit of eating the donkeys in the end!

> The solution for the lions is to lead and not to be led. An appetite for donkey flesh is however not to be discouraged.

11

References

1 Mintzberg. *The Rise and Fall of Strategic Planning.* Hemel Hempstead: Prentice Hall, 1994.
2 Luke S. *Power. a Radical View.* London: Macmillan, 1974.
3 Lee-Potter J. *A Damn Bad Business.* London: Gollancz, 1997.
4 Coulson J. Doctors under stress. *BMA News Rev* 1996;April:22–6.
5 Karpur N, Borrill C, Stride C. Psychological morbidity and job satisfaction in hospital consultants and junior house officers. *Br Med J* 1998;**317**:511–12.
6 Ramirez AJ *et al.* Mental health of hospital consultants: the effects of stress and job satisfaction at work. *Lancet* 1996;**347**:724–8.
7 Spurgeon P, Barwell F, Maxwell R. Types of work stress and the implications for the role of general practitioners. *Health Serv Management Res* 1995;**8**:186–97.
8 Allen I. *Doctors and their Careers.* London: Policy Studies Institute, 1994, p. 229.
9 Kendall RE, Pearce A. Consultant psychiatrists who retired prematurely in 1995 and 1996. *Psychol Bull* 1997;**21**:741–5.
10 Illich I. *Medical Nemesis: the Expropriation of Health.* Calder and Boyars, 1975.
11 Harrison R, Pollitt C. *Controlling Health Professionals.* Milton Keynes: Open University Press, 1994, pp. 2–3.
12 Hadley R, Forster D, eds. *Doctors as Managers.* London: Longmans, 1986, p. 162 *et seq.*
13 Friedson E. *Profession of Medicine: a Study of the Sociology of Applied Knowledge.* London: Harper and Row, 1970.
14 Turner BS. *Medical Power and Social Knowledge.* London: Sage, 1987, chap. 7.
15 *Report of the NHS Management Enquiry.* London: DHSS, 1983.
16 *Health Care UK 1996/7.* London: The King's Fund, 1997, p. 2.
17 Micklethwait J, Wooldridge A. *The Witch Doctors.* London: Mandarin, 1997, p. 341.
18 Lee-Potter J. *A Damn Bad Business.* London: Gollancz, 1997, p. 242.

2 Starting up as a Medical Manager

Before you accept a medical management post there are questions to ask yourself:

- Do I want to do it and why?
- Am I the right age?
- What will the job involve?
- Do I have the necessary skills?
- How do I prepare myself?

2.1 Do I want to do it?

We can subdivide this question into three:

(1) Do you want to do it as an end in itself?
(2) Or as a means to an end?
(3) Or as a simple professional obligation for its own sake, or because you have been dragooned or flattered into it?

Few people enter medical management because they wish it to be the main focus of the rest of their professional lives, and I suspect most go in as a category three prisoner simply because they feel they ought to. They do not do it resentfully and the prospect will probably interest them. By contrast, it is worth mentioning that there are some disreputable reasons for going in which may help you in making your decision. For example, "I don't want anyone else to do the job", "I don't believe anyone can do the job as well as I can", "I want to have power over my colleagues", or, "I want to use it as a vehicle to get what I want from the organisation". Alternatively, perhaps you are a "control freak"—a much overused term which I take to mean that you need to have a finger in every pie, to have everything possible under your control. Okay, but why the "freak" suffix? I don't recall that

13

Napoleon or Wellington were exceptionally freakish in the gangly, slightly loony use of the word.

You must not be under any illusion that it will make you popular. In this context you can bear in mind the Congolese proverb "the higher up the tree the monkey climbs the more his bottom shows" or more politely quote yourself Luke, chapter VII, verse I "It needs must be that offences come, but woe unto those through whom they come". Lastly, do not expect to do it to make money. It may increase your salary a bit and if you do it well it just might help you in the merit award stakes, but rarely enough to offset the hassles.

You will need to have a moderately rounded personality, for the successful manager needs a diversity of traits and skills if the job is to be done adequately—interpersonal skills of course, an ability to collate and react to information, the ability to plan and to implement the plan. I must confess to enjoying planning but like much less the hard grind of execution. I have discovered that this is not merely my problem, it is widespread, and managers often enjoy the planning which should be 10% of the effort but are much less enthralled by the other 90% of effort that needs next to be expended on execution.

2.2 Am I the right age?

The correct age for appointment to a clinical management post is often debated and there is no right answer. It is however good practice for young clinicians to look at their possible future career path before accepting a management post. Clinical director posts are time consuming and reduce the opportunities for developing or practising other skills. Furthermore, when a clinician has spent a few years in a management post she has learned a set of skills and obtained a body of knowledge that makes her a very valuable asset to the organisation. . .but only if she continues in management. The consequence is that some young clinicians become "trapped" into a sequence of management posts from which they may emerge too late to develop other possibly more rewarding avenues of personal development. We need young clinicians in management for their vigour, open mindedness and longevity, but the potential damage to the full breadth of an individual's career needs to be considered and discussed openly before appointment. Senior jobs such as medical director and executive committee member may be more appropriate for the older, more streetwise clinician. The actual ages of 702 clinical directors who responded to a British Association of Medical Managers (BAMM) survey is shown in Figure 2.1.

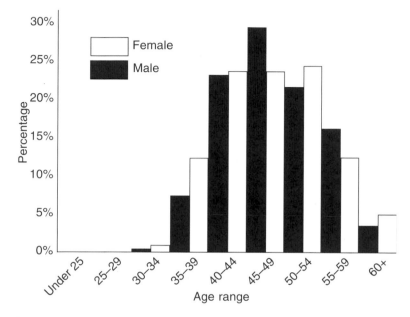

Figure 2.1   Age spectrum of clinical directors. (Data source: British Association of Medical Managers, 1997)

2.3 Do I have the skills?

You certainly must not think that because you were intelligent and laborious enough to qualify as a doctor that you can automatically slip into management and be good at it. Also you must not think that because your clinical firm works well you thereby have the skills needed to run a more complex business with a less well defined hierarchy.

Insofar as personal qualities are concerned you will be helped by having:

- *Patience*—which includes tolerating long waits to see things happen.
- *Resilience*—willingness to put up with repeated frustrations.

15

- *Perspicacity*—the ability to see the wood in spite of all the trees.
- *Leadership* skills.

You will also need some practical skills, chief among which I would include:

- The ability to read amounts of exceptionally boring paperwork at times when you are tired and yet be able to extract the crucial facts from it.
- The ability to understand the work and attitudes of people not normally in your ambit.
- Time management—I have to confess that this was something I personally never managed, indeed I even failed to find the time to attend the one-day time management course which had been booked for me!

2.3.1 Leadership skills

I suspect most people believe that leaders are born and not made and that, furthermore, charismatic heroes existed in history. They might therefore believe that in smaller environments there must be those imbued with smaller versions of these skills of leadership and equally those that are bereft of them. Historians have searched for the skills that mark off great leaders from other mortals and no biography is complete without that sort of analysis, but the skills do not seem to be common between leaders. Modern social science fashion takes the antiheroic view that leadership depends more on context and is dependent on the character of the followers and the particular situation to hand rather than to any special powers that a leader might have. Churchill for example was an excellent wartime leader but an unremarkable peacetime leader. Leadership in the powerful, directive sense is simply unfashionable in this age of passive liberalism. The autonomy of little groups is considered to be the mainspring of productive work and they need to be "facilitated" rather than directed. The age of the intermediary is indeed upon us[1] and the manager has become the true intermediary, functioning primarily as a catalyst. For the medical manager this is important because fashionably his leadership is supposed to be through quiet influencing rather than through rabble-rousing oratory or a publicly glamorous leadership persona. Leadership will need to be through example, particularly in the style of his or her clinical performance. However persuasive the medical manager's tongue, it is unlikely that colleagues will be persuaded to accept a rule or a change if he fails openly to accept them himself. Leadership is, after all, a mutual relationship between the leader and the led, in which the leader must balance three crucial components: The Task ... The Team ... and The Individual.

In spite of this seeming absence of overt leadership characteristics, someone will no doubt have spotted some old-fashioned leadership skills in you before offering you a management job, so you do not need to be on the lookout for a course or a book on leadership skills—you may already have them. In 1513 Machiavelli the first management guru wrote "The Prince" as a leadership course for Duke Lorenzo the Magnificent of Florence, but the Duke felt it was unnecessary for someone already confidently in post, preferring a pair of hunting dogs given to him at the same time by another suitor. He would probably have supported Lord Sheppard's view of leadership as "Management by a light grip on the throat".

Incidentally, I believe we do have some need for heroic leaders in the NHS, for grey is indeed the colour of management. The red heat of conflict and the purple of passion are not currently welcomed in the NHS manager—perhaps they should be! There should be in the NHS what Peters describes as "preachers of vision".[2] Their moment will return because today's truths of management theory are quickly supplanted by tomorrow's or even yesterday's, because one of the features of this sort of social science is that there are no testable truths so your guess about how best to manage is probably as good as theirs, or mine. If management theory did not change management gurus would quickly be bereft of something to publish and have no revolutionary message with which to "theme" expensive seminars ... They would also be unemployed.

2.4 What does it involve? How will I prepare myself?

Too many people enter medical management without a very clear idea of what will be asked of them and therefore not knowing whether they can deliver effectively. Some homework is therefore needed before you accept the job. The next chapter outlines what it is that medical managers do, but you will need to make sure that your particular job is defined before you accept it. If you read no other section of this book I would suggest that this is the crucial bit.

17

You need to be happy that five areas have been dealt with:

(1) That you have an explicit role.
(2) That you have an explicit contract.
(3) That explicit training is available.
(4) That explicit clinical back-up arrangements have been made.
(5) That explicit arrangements for re-entry into the clinical world at end of job have been made.

2.4.1 An explicit role

Ask the following questions:

(1) What area will I be managing?
(2) What managerial support will I have?
(3) What will be my relationship to the managerial support? Do they work for me or do I work for them?
(4) What office support will be available? Check that the extra work will not merely devolve onto your already overloaded clinical secretary.
(5) What will be my relationship with nursing staff? Is there a nurse manager and what is our professional relationship?
(6) What are my reporting lines? Am I answerable directly to the chief executive, to the medical director or to some other medical or non-medical manager?

You should make sure that you have all these in the form of a letter, or at least you should write it down following the first meeting to discuss the job. Clinical directors and medical directors should have an explicit job description, though in our trust we have tried to get away from the convoluted, detailed job description to a more general one. The Association of Trust Medical Directors[3] has produced an excellent publication outlining in a wider way the responsibilities of a medical director, and although not many medical directors have the strength to take on all those tasks, the document should at least be read before the job is accepted. The type of tasks that a medical manager undertakes are implicit in the contents of this book but more explicit in Sections 3.1 and 4.8

18

2.4.2 An explicit contract

More questions to ask:

(1) How many notional half-days am I expected to work at this?
(2) Will they count as fixed or unfixed sessions?
(3) What is the term of my job?
(4) What notice should I give or can I be given?
(5) What is the remuneration? Is this an honorarium or is it superannuable?
(6) Is there access to a budget for training and for professional travel?
(7) Will I be expected to sign a confidentiality clause? Most doctors find such clauses to be anathema and most would probably refuse to sign one. They should not be necessary. If your trust demands one in your contract, make sure that it applies only to genuinely "commercial" issues and not to professional judgments you might make about the care patients are receiving. Gagging you from speaking out about what you believe to be the proper care of patients is to infringe your professional rights as a doctor. Fortunately the Minister of Health announced in October 1997 that "gagging clauses" would be outlawed in future contracts.[4] Additionally there will be the provisions of clinical governance and the right to speak out in good faith will be enshrined in a Public Interest Disclosure bill which is likely to become law in 1999.
(8) If my sessions are to be added to my NHS sessions and so bring them up to full time, will I still be entitled to undertake private practice if I wish?
(9) What is my budget, who sets it and who reviews it?
(10) Is there PRP (performance related payment)?

2.4.3 Explicit training

Whether you need any training prior to taking up your appointment really depends on you and your experience. It is difficult in prospect to know which of your skills will be deficient when it comes to management. Many clinical directors have come into post and functioned excellently with no prior management training whatsoever. There are a number of readable and relevant books outlining the practical management knowledge that a clinical director might need, and some are listed at the end of this chapter. Membership of the British Association of Medical Managers and, if you are a medical director, the Association of Trust Medical Directors is, I would say, mandatory and attendance at their conferences or some of their short courses would probably suffice for most people. I would like to think that the skills required of a good manager are human skills or quickly learnt by an intelligent, open minded clinician. If there is formal training which she needs it is about the mechanics of management within the Health Service; how the finances work, how decisions are made, how purchasing is undertaken and so forth. These are listed in section 4.8 "Professional development". I personally have an aversion to formal training in management skills, but I must be in a minority because this is a boom industry in the Health Service as elsewhere. Courses in management training, seminars on current issues and mini-conferences abound. As a medical director I received between five and ten announcements for such events in my mail each week, most with glossy, persuasive blurbs puffed out with pictures of the lecturers and selected quotes from contented attenders at previous courses. The common feature of the courses seem to be that one has never heard of 90% of the speakers, 90% are more expensive than seems reasonable on any judgment, 90% have been set up for purely commercial reasons, 90% of the content of each course seems to be of no immediate relevance to one's real job. As a consequence I quickly reached the point where 90% of such announcements went straight into my wastepaper basket. Reading the pundits you would think that educational information about practical management skills was something new. Anyone who believes that should perhaps read the "Meditations" of Marcus Aurelius written in the second century AD; for example book VI number 50:

> try to move men by persuasion not against their will if the principles of justice so direct. But if someone uses force to obstruct you, then take a different line; resign yourself without a pang and turn the obstacle into an opportunity for the exercise in some other virtue.

The NHS has an unfortunate habit of trying to mimic today what happened in business the day before yesterday. The present obsession with business management courses is symptomatic of this although their relevance and effectiveness within the NHS remains untested. Nevertheless, fashion dictates that sending new clinical directors to an expensive country hotel to role play and put up tents blindfold will make things better.

The sceptic will note that the motive for "sending clinicians off on a management course" is frequently not a desire to make them good, practical managers but to inculcate in them an understanding of what managers have to do, and why they have to do it. It is hoped that afterwards the clinician will be more cooperative, or at least sympathetic. That of course is an entirely proper motive but it is probably more sensible to start working towards that particular educational objective at the undergraduate stage, though very discreetly.

While you may not need any formal training, you will certainly need to set aside time for a formal period of induction in which you spend some time with the major players in the organisation generally and in your area in particular. You must also physically visit each ward, office, outpatient clinic, etc. for which you will have responsibility and ensure that the staff there know your name and your face. It is extraordinary how bad doctors are at arranging such induction time—usually pleading shortage of time. This induction period is too important to skimp, and it may save you a lot of time later, also it is a good introduction to the skill of MBWA (Management By Walking Around).

Books on management theory and the MBA
Bookshops, especially those at airports and stations, have large sections devoted to books about management: "The Way to Win", "Think and Grow Rich", "The Foundations of Corporate Success", "A Passion for Excellence", "The One Minute Manager", and so on. About $750 million worth of books about business is sold every year in the USA alone, and they are less addicted to them than the British. Many of these titles have made their authors millionaires, but it is claimed very few are read from end to end. Managers' anxiety not to be outflanked by a new idea continues to sell these books, while faddism and the lack of objective ways of judging their worth guarantees a steady flow of new books. If you are minded to buy one first read Micklethwait and Wooldridge's book *The Witch Doctors*. These editors of *The Economist* have appraised all the management gurus' texts and present the case both for them and against. They summarise the general case against management theorising thus:[5]

21

- It is constitutionally incapable of self criticism.
- Its terminology usually confuses rather than educates.
- It rarely rises above common sense.
- It is faddish and bedevilled by contradictions that would not be allowed in more rigorous disciplines.

That said they sometimes make interesting reading when you have a particular problem to hand, but are usually only worth dipping into. What you must not do is believe them. The bestselling management book, Peter's "In Search of Excellence"[6] analysed the factors that led to the success of a cohort of American businesses and exhorted others to copy them. Unfortunately, two-thirds of those top companies have now fallen from grace. You will probably find something more sustaining elsewhere in the bookshop.

The MBA (Master of Business Administration) is sometimes floated past clinical managers as a "good thing to do". I really think it is inappropriate unless you have quite considerable experience in clinical management and envisage your future in it. Even then it may be a waste of time, the MBA is after all sometimes lampooned by senior managers as "MBA, Maybe Best Avoided". In the USA 75 000 MBAs are awarded each year. In the UK currently a hundred institutions offer MBAs and the part-time courses last between 2 and 5 years. They are expensive, costing up to £20 000, and place enormous pressure on the participant to devote his spare time and energy to the course. Even in the business world there is now considerable doubt as to the value of the MBA and although in management interviews the candidates' possession of the MBA may get them onto the short-list, I have been struck by how little attention is paid to it during the actual business of selection. Forty per cent of people with MBAs leave their company within a year of getting the MBA, in two cases out of three this is said to be due to the employer failing to reward the possession of an MBA; this occurs especially in the public sector.[7] In fairness one should, however, add that many managers said that it was a seminal intellectual event in their lives and felt that the effort was well worth while.

2.4.4 Explicit clinical back-up arrangements

Unless you are under-employed you cannot take on any significant clinical management role without giving up some clinical work. At first sight it may seem that this will not be necessary, but I and many other clinical managers have learnt by bitter experience that clinical management can never happen as an add-on role. It must be an explicit part of your timetable. For this reason before accepting any clinical management post you will need to examine your clinical timetable and discuss with the chief executive or medical director how the necessary space is to be freed up in your timetable. This may require you dropping some sessions, colleagues may need to take up these sessions or it may even be necessary to appoint new clinical staff to take on the work. If either of the latter happen you must make absolutely certain, in writing, that those sessions will revert to you when you complete your term in clinical management.

2.4.5 "Re-entry" arrangements

It is very easy to get caught up in the business of clinical management to the neglect of your clinical practice and your continuing clinical education. You will, in addition, almost certainly have given up some clinical work to enable you to be a clinical manager. These factors can make it quite difficult to re-enter clinical practice smoothly at the end of your time in management, and unless the necessary arrangements have been made in advance you may even be trapped into a situation where you may not wish to remain in clinical management long term but it becomes your predominant skill. I would suggest, therefore, that at the outset of your appointment to a clinical management post you ensure that it is explicit and in writing that when you return to your clinical post you will have the same number of sessions to return to and that some arrangements will be made to allow whatever re-training is necessary. My trust is both far seeing and generous in that it allows senior clinical managers sabbatical leave of 3 months after 3 or more years in post and pays for attendance at courses etc. during that sabbatical leave. That seems to me to be a proper way of managing these things and ought to be the norm for all NHS trusts, though most will not be able to afford it.

2.5 How much will I be paid?

In 1997 the Fitzhugh Directory of NHS Trusts revealed that the Medical Director of St Mary's was earning an annual salary of

£43 000 in addition to his clinical salary of £88 000 and whatever he was earning in his private practice. This is untypically high but still chickenfeed next to the $million salaries of medical directors in the USA and substantially more than most clinicians in management can expect.

Most are paid the equivalent of one or two clinical sessions.

2.6 Conclusion

You will have noted that I have assumed in this chapter that you will be moving into medical management and then, in due course, out of it back into your original clinical role. It is probable that you will slip in and out of management over your career, but on current evidence fewer than 10% of clinical managers will stay on in medical management as a long term major activity, and only a handful will give up their clinical work to become full-time managers, if only because most must have realised that to do so would lose them their "street credibility". Because of this tangential relationship with management it is of critical importance for the clinician, before she embarks on this route, to view it as if she were the pilot of an untried aeroplane. "Am I sufficiently trained for this flight?", "Is the vehicle in which I am flying air-worthy?", "What will happen to me during the flight?" and "Have sufficient preparations been made for me to make a smooth landing?" The use of that simple analogy could spare you and your institution a lot of heartache.

Helpful books on clinical management
Hansell M, Salter B, eds. *The Clinician's Management Handbook.* London: Saunders, 1995.

Hirst DK, Clements RV. *Clinical Directors' Handbook.* London: Churchill Livingstone, 1995.

Lees P, ed. *Navigating the NHS.* Oxford: BAMM, Radcliffe Medical Press, 1996.

Riley J. *Helping Doctors who Manage: Learning from Experience.* London: King's Fund Publishing, 1998.

Simpson J, Smith R, eds. *Management for Doctors.* London: BMJ Publishing Group, 1995.

References

1 Zeldin T. *An Intimate History of Mankind.* London: Minerva, 1995, pp. 147–65.

2 Peters T. *Thriving on Chaos*. London: Macmillan, 1987.
3 Association of Trust Medical Directors. *The Role and Responsibilities of the Medical Director*. 1996.
4 *Br Med J* 1997;**315**:836.
5 Micklethwait J, Wooldridge A. *The Witch Doctors*. London: Mandarin, 1997, p. 15.
6 Peters T, Waterman R. *In Search of Excellence: Lessons from America's Best Run Companies*. New York: Harper & Row, 1982.
7 Welch J. *People Management* 1997;**3**:12.

3 The Medical Manager's Work

3.1 What do medical managers do?

3.1.1 Introduction

This chapter concerns itself with what medical managers actually do and, to a lesser extent, with what they ought to do. This latter twist is, however, more fully dealt with in Section 4.8 on professional development. It was noted at the outset that medical management includes a wide range of roles, including educational roles, such as clinical tutor and postgraduate dean. The titles of those appointed to mainstream management positions in trusts range from lead clinician, chief or chairman of the department, service director, head of division, etc., but more than 80% are called clinical director. The job of medical director is an explicitly different one.

3.1.2 Clinical director

The information on what clinical directors actually do is derived primarily from a British Association of Medical Managers' (BAMM) survey published in 1997.[1] That survey found that most clinical directors work 2.5–5 sessions at management tasks (the average being 3.12), but the average contracted time is 1.62 (i.e. 1 or 2 sessions). Therefore most clinical directors can expect to work for twice as long as the contract predicts. Eighty-four per cent manage a budget and that budget ranges from £50 000 to £20 million. The commonest is £2–3 million. Contentiously, though, this is usually not the whole budget for the clinical director's area of responsibility. In particular it tends to exclude information technology, capital items, equipment replacement, nursing, recruitment, and theatre services. Having said that, of the 69% of clinical directors providing a list of principal items in their budget, the order of frequency of mentioning items was as follows:

- hospital
- staff salaries
- pharmacy/drugs
- disposable/consumables
- equipment and its maintenance
- computers and IT consumables
- support services
- capital charges
- training and education.

It is an interesting aside in the document that although 66% of clinical directors were able to use savings generated in their budget, 34% were not, which is hardly a stimulus to a commitment to budgetary prudence.

When it comes to summarising clinical directors' roles, one study has abbreviated those roles as:

- budget management
- business planning
- corporate decision making
- overall clinical and service direction
- quality assurance
- staff management.

or more prosaically as:

- appoint clinical and support staff
- define and negotiate contracts
- purchase equipment
- quality issues and the handling of complaints
- staff disciplinary procedures
- strategic planning
- whole or partial responsibility for directorate budget.[2]

These jobs divide themselves into housekeeping tasks such as personnel, budget details and purchasing, for which the clinical director should oversee the tasks for which his clinical knowledge is important and which cannot be done as well by a non-clinical manager. This will be especially the areas of defining the directorate strategy using his clinical knowledge of the directorate. He is

27

particularly well placed in this to determine what actions within the directorate can be taken to exploit strengths and support weaknesses. It is also necessary for the clinical director to be involved in negotiating with purchasers to ensure realistic and achievable contracts are entered into and to decide which areas need quality improvement and indeed, to lead in that improvement. Lastly the clinical director needs to be able to sense when New Deal and Calman training targets are not being met, in spite of what is said to him and to act accordingly.

There are some areas which clinical directors are edged into, and you will need to take your own counsel as to whether they are proper tasks.

One area is the details of *contracting* which is a highly complex area. While you need to understand the difference between different types of contract such as "Block" and "Cost and Volume", and to understand the impact of these on your directorate's function, you should fundamentally be merely supporting rather than leading the process.

Another difficult area is *marketing*. This popped onto the agenda in the wake of the market-style reforms of the Health Service that came with "Working for Patients" and quickly began to appear as chapters in books on medical management (chapters almost never written by doctors). Marketing as a concept means different things to different people, but to most of us it implies not simple provision of what is requested but actively selling a product. In this case the product is a skill, and actively selling means going beyond what is asked of you as a provider, and attempting to create a market. Apologists will say that marketing is in fact all about researching what the public wants, tailoring your product to their needs. That is not, I think, what the general public understands by marketing. We get into difficult areas here. Clinical teams with specialist skills may wish to attract patients and may even produce "advertising" material to underpin and communicate the pride in their service. However there is a narrow line between this and the aggressive unit-against-unit marketing which began to be a feature of some units emboldened by the market reforms of "Working for Patients". What is important is that the clinical director is aware of the constructive features of this communications exercise in marketing and makes sure that the facts that underpin the advertising are available when debates take place with the purchasers. An exception perhaps is where a service needs more patients to function optimally and so the clinical director may need to actively go out to new purchasers and perhaps to look for that work. In the current style of the NHS though these things should be part of a sensible, cooperative negotiation about rationalisation and location of services and not a "go get it", winners and losers kind of approach. But you may disagree with me about this.

Clinical directors do what they do largely for historic reasons; put crudely doctors needed to do the dirty managerial jobs to bring them to their economic senses and to use them as agents to control their colleagues and thus the budget. We ought to have grown out of this now, although the BAMM study still reports that most clinical directors feel used, undervalued, and not part of their organisation's core decision making processes. Too many are also involved in straightforward managerial chores that any manager could do (possibly better). The point has been made that we are an under-doctored country and cannot afford to lose so many top clinicians to management posts—doctors who should have their shoulders to the clinical wheel. Their time in management should therefore be used efficiently, this means an increased strategic role and allocating them adequate administrative clerical and managerial support. Unfortunately in order to let doctors into the central part of the decision-making process many of the organisations will need to change their "closed-door" culture.

3.1.3 How does real life match up to this?

Once, tired of counting sheep, I got up and wrote down the problems that were currently taxing me as a clinical director. The list went as follows (it is not prioritised):

- New Deal hours—Still not working, need to employ phlebotomists and nurse practitioners. On what budget?
- Calman—Still no consultant sessions dedicated to this. Needs more sessions. Needs more budget.
- Continuity of care.
- Nurse recruitment—Need to fund yet another overseas trawl.
- Alcoholic Mr X—Still need written evidence.
- Purchasers want higher percentage day-case surgery—Need paper to indicate difficulties of this in our deprived catchment area.

29

- Insufficient beds—Medical outliers as ever. No prospect of cross-subsidy.
- Radiology cross-charging—Up again due to "research activity".
- Study leave—Excessive and uncontrollable for academics, still no funding though for junior study leave.
- Complaint—MP still harassing us over a purely vexatious claim. Doesn't know the facts but expects action of some sort.
- Short-listing for consultant anaesthetist (again).
- MRSA (again).
- Stocking problem—Too many different hip prostheses. Need to persuade consultants to use a smaller range.
- Waiting-list computer software—Problems (again).
- List of audit projects for purchaser—Needed this week but no reply about last year's yet. Need to persuade them to compare same projects from different providers.
- Finance director—Still asking for £400k out of the budget!
- Prepare talk for management development seminar.
- Respond to Specialist Advisory Committee (SAC) document summarising their visit.

And those were just the directorate's problems and excluded trustwide issues.

It is said that the good manager can deal with a maximum of five problems at a time. Ideally she should ask her personal assistant to type them onto a small card, which is kept handy in a suit pocket for ready reference. It is not like that. But perhaps therein lies the buzz of management and the real message should be not so much that there should be five problems but that the effective manager should be solving no more than five problems at any one time.

3.1.4 The medical director

Medical director is a statutory post on the trust's board and as such is not the same as the old post of medical superintendent nor, it must be stressed, is the director the consultant's representative on a trust board. He is appointed by the chairman and non-executive directors of the board with the chief executive's advice. Although he is not the representative of clinicians in the trust, it would be foolish to appoint someone who did not carry the approval of the consultant body.

Once appointed the medical director is a full and equivalent member of the board, he is a director of the trust and, as such, has a peer relationship with the chief executive and other board members and shares with them a corporate responsibility for policy and decision making within the trust and the shaping of objectives. The medical director is managerially responsible to the board and is not the chairman's or the chief executive's medical poodle. He is less a prisoner of the status quo than is the clinical director.

Just as all executive members of the board have specific responsibilities, so too does the medical director. His responsibilities are not statutorily defined and will vary from trust to trust. The wide range of those tasks has been defined in a document produced by the Association of Trust Medical Directors in 1996, which enquired of more than 250 medical directors what their roles were.[3] The list it produced is too onerous to be achieved by any one medical director; a better summary is the generic one produced by the Central Consultants and Specialists Committee in their document "CCSC Guidance for Developing the Role of Medical Directors". They identified core tasks of the medical director as:

- Providing professional medical advice to the trust board and its officers.
- Providing medical input to the development of strategy and strategic thinking.
- Communicating the trust perspective to clinicians.
- Supporting the work and development of clinical directors.
- Taking a key role in doctors' disciplinary procedures.
- Taking part in the management of investigations of a clinical nature concerning doctors, such as arise from complaints or untoward events.
- Taking part in consultant appointment procedures and discretionary points and merit award systems.

To these should be added the recent issue of the overseeing of clinical governance.

In all of these the medical director needs to be more than just a doctor. He needs to develop new and different networks from those he had as a doctor and to bring in ideas for clinicians from outside their normal milieu. These tasks will probably occupy at least five sessions a week. Whereas the clinical directors are appointed by a range of mechanisms from chief executive's whim to Buggin's turn, the process of appointing a medical director is much more defined and properly should be advertised and interviews held with representatives from the board present who will have taken soundings. Medical directors should be respected as, or at least credible to, clinicians and therefore ought not to be full-time medical directors. Neither should they concurrently be clinical directors so as to avoid clashes of priority or of obligation. As with clinical directors there is a risk that they will become bogged down in mundane issues requiring no clinical input. It is crucial that there is appropriate managerial and administrative support.

For the medical director as for the clinical director the trick is to escape from the jobs that are merely "housekeeping" and try to concentrate on the tasks that support improvement and innovation, and to make these not just reactive but visionary, looking beyond the obvious next step.

3.2 Nurses and management

The two great professions of medicine are doctoring and nursing. Traditionally they worked together in a comprehensible, synergistic way doing different tasks but with the doctor recognised as the dominant partner. Many of us have spent the majority of our professional lives in this environment in which it is accepted that the doctor is the clinical decision maker. This relationship between doctors and nurses has however changed and continues to change with no clear end in sight. The changes are important for medical managers for four reasons:

(1) Nurses form the greatest part of the hospital workforce.
(2) Their management by doctors is a contentious area.
(3) Because healthcare can only be delivered effectively when doctors and nurses work together with clearly identified roles.
(4) Because the national and increasing shortage of nurses will force changes in the pattern of what they do.

So without apology there follows a brief history lesson on changes in nursing which have occurred over the past 30 years, because without that the present stresses and changes in nursing cannot be understood by the medical manager. For the detail I am primarily indebted to Rivett's account of the history of the NHS.[4]

3.2.1 The development of nursing

Although the profession of nursing arose as much from a reaction against the drunken slatterns who supervised the filthy inmates of hospital wards before the end of the nineteenth century as it did from dedicated religious orders of earlier times, it is to the latter that we owe the concept of service that was formalised into a moral framework. To most people, nursing still represents a vocational ideal and, until recently, the attributes of the nurse were always considered to be those of "dedication, kindness, compassion, patience, trustworthiness, self-control, discretion, humility, perseverance, courtesy, the obedience of loyalty and respect".[5] Inherent in this position were not just huge status, but also low pay, subservience to doctors and even depersonalisation to an extent. Until recently ward sisters at St Thomas' were known by their ward and had no names of their own. This sounded fine when there were nice ward names and you could be called Sister Alexandra or Sister Florence but it depersonalised the sister and, anyway, it did not have quite the same ring when you were called Sister X-ray or Sister Gynae. Outpatients.

The status was stable from the time of Florence Nightingale until the 1960s when both society and hospital practice began to change. Nursing came to be seen as a temporary job with high recruitment and high wastage, and the hospitals' shortened stay and increased dependency significantly increased the pressures of working as a nurse. Until the 1960s education for nurses had been seen primarily as a practical activity to be undertaken at the bedside, apart from some theoretical knowledge passed on by medical staff. From the 1960s a desire for a more explicit education for nurses came to the fore and nursing education for the right or the wrong reasons became more and more to resemble the education of medical students; indeed from now on it is likely that much nursing and medical student education at the undergraduate level will be undertaken jointly.

Nursing was and still is predominantly a female profession. In the 1960s women's rights and feminism were abroad. Education was seen as liberation and specifically in this case was identified as freedom from the shackles of primarily male doctors and from the passive role of selfless service and caring that reflected discredited domestic roles. The propaganda for women was that this kind of activity was no longer to be seen as rewarding or appropriate. The development of nursing was increasingly led by educationalists and the theories that drove them mostly came from over the Atlantic. In May 1986 the proposals that were to become Project 2000 were lodged. Project 2000 was to transform the nature of student nursing such that the student was no longer educated on the ward, no longer a pair of hands while being educated. The legacy of Florence Nightingale was at last defunct and, in spite of government anxiety about the cost and staffing implications of Project 2000, it was accepted and it was envisaged at the same moment that the hands-on work of patient care would in many ways be replaced by a new grade of support workers. Nursing in a professional and educational sense had changed but had to some extent gained a power to fashion its own direction, and what we have seen since then is experimental and theoretical attempts going in many different directions, some frustrating and most confusing the watcher, and indeed many confusing nurses themselves.

The developments occurring in nursing have been fuelled by inescapable changes in healthcare such as higher patient turn-over, higher dependency, the need for discharge planning, the empowerment of patients, quality assessment exercises and the disappearance of social workers from the wards. Unfortunately, the fact that many of the changes have been dressed up in educationalist, socialist or feminist political jargon has not helped. New concepts have involved "team nursing", the concept of "the named nurse". These fragmented the original cohesive concept of the ward which doctors recognised as working so well. The concept of "the nursing process" was imported from the USA and required a formal and systematic review and documentation of patients' needs and a plan for dealing with them—"The Care Plan". Nurses developed paperwork of their own, running parallel to the doctor's clinical record, and doctors noticed that nurses spent more time writing or in huddles around Sister's desk than at the bedside. Nursing had begun to run in parallel to medicine.

The upheaval in nursing did, to the enormous benefit of healthcare, spawn nurses who were able to practice independently in a way that previously only midwives and district nurses had done: the nurse specialist, the nurse practitioner, nurse counsellors, independent midwives, etc. By this time the Royal College of Nursing was able to admit that not only was nursing separate from medicine in its day-to-day care of patients, but even accepted that nursing goals might differ from clinical goals. Many nurses found this empowering. Many found it deeply worrying, but whichever of these you believed an unfortunate side-effect, as Rivett has noted, is that the distance politically between doctors and nurses was widening at a time when they needed to be cohesive to resist outside threats to patient care.

3.2.2 Nursing and management

It was at the upper end of the nursing hierarchy that the change was most profound and for medical managers the ramifications of those changes are most important to understand and to empathise with.

Before the 1970s the shape of the nursing hierarchy was absolutely clear. Matron was in change, "her" ward sisters were responsible to her, the ward nurses were responsible to sister. A neat comprehensible and functional family unit: but society has changed. Hospital is no longer the focus for a nurse's life. Turnover has increased, loyalty has wavered and this cosy family structure has apparently become no longer appropriate. Additionally, there was a continuing problem of no real career spaces between ward sister and matron. The shortages of senior posts at this level made it difficult for nurses to influence the overall management of hospitals, and many nurses never achieved promotion beyond sister grade and the relatively inadequate salaries that those attracted.

The Salmon Report of 1966 inserted tiers of nursing administration above sister, the old concept of matron as a kind of "Mother Superior" figure disappeared and the involvement of nurses in management as the only way to a higher salary was established. In management matters they had several heads' start over the doctors, whose influence at this stage was still by committee. Nurses trained themselves in management but their management only ran to the management of nurses, they never really got a grip on the central power base of hospitals or of the Health Service. Griffiths, the author of the Griffiths Report of 1983, which brought in the concept of general management, is said to have regarded nurses as "doe-eyed and dangerous" and his reforms left nurses with no meaningful role. They have continued to exist in the shadows of non-clinical administrators and managers and even though directors of nursing sit at the top table as full board members, their salaries are scandalously lower than those of their managerial peers around the table and their powers very constrained.

When clinical management structures began to evolve in the wake of the Griffiths Report, the directorates that were set up often had one or more nurse managers. However, to this day it is unclear whether the intention was for nurse managers to manage the nurses or just to be managers who happened also to be nurses.

The common sense arrangement which can apply in clinical directorates is a triumvirate of managers: a doctor manager, a nurse manager, and a non-clinical manager. The situation has however now evolved to a point where, as best one can judge, many nurses who are managers are accepted as equivalent to any other manager but whose special skills happen to be in nursing just as another manager's might be in personnel or finance. In this arrangement the doctor medical manager is often potentially in a difficult position in relation to the nurses in the directorate. It may be that they are technically under his "command", yet at the same time they remain professionally accountable to matron's successor, the director of nursing, and in the midst of this is the nurse manager who is uncomfortably seated part way between the clinical director and the director of nursing. The nurse in that role may find her role potentially compromised by having to satisfy two separate agendas: the professional development of nurses and their responsibility to the patients as one-to-one carers while at the same time satisfying a management agenda that may wish to look critically at nursing establishment, nursing practices, etc. This is the same difficult position as a clinical director can find himself in, and in fact it should encourage both the clinical director and the nurse manager to share their difficulties and their solutions. The position of nurses on the executive of trusts is no easier. A Royal College of Nursing study carried out in 1996 surveyed 340 nurse executive directors.[6] The report showed that these executives, trust board members, had a large range of job titles, 56 in total, yet interestingly less than a quarter were responsible for managing nursing services. The tendency was for them to manage low-budget areas without line management responsibilities. As alluded to above their salaries are lower than those of other board members. Half those surveyed said they were the lowest paid board member—25% wanted to leave, 47% wanted to change their jobs within the next 2 years and only 14% wanted to stay on until retirement.

In view of the numerical size of the nursing workforce, its increasing level of education, both undergraduate and post-graduate, its commitment to change and to managerial training, it is depressing that nurses have not yet established a larger role in the machinery of the Health Service. One can only hope that this will improve in the future. As far as the individual medical manager is concerned, his starting point when establishing a relationship with the nurse in management is to realise that the nurse will probably be the closest to him in terms of professional instincts and is a natural ally. The medical manager must, however, bear in mind that all is not well in the world of nursing. To quote Ann Bradshaw:[5]

> a split has formed between graduate nurses and vocational nurses who carry out practical tasks. Elitist nursing, intellectually unable to convince healthcare reformers of the need for advanced nursing practice, has alienated the vocational and practical majority of nurses...UK nursing theory has displaced plain and simple caring, but not for a hard, technical science akin to medicine. Rather, social science dominates academic nursing knowledge and technique. Art and science have both been displaced and deconstructed, but is this breakdown beneficial for the care of patients? In the primary interest of patients, an informed, dispassionate and rational debate is needed in the public arena to consider the nature and purpose of nursing and nurse training.

There are a lot of issues here that managers need to deal with; not just the dangers of gender politics but also the practical ones of a demoralised, under-rewarded, underempowered group right at the heart of the organisation. Somehow a career structure has to be found that incorporates the old loving habits of bedside nursing, meaningful incorporation in the wider management of the service and a career development programme that does not depend at its upper end on the achievement of yet more classroom-based qualifications.

3.3 Committees

Committees are the life-blood of oligarchic management, but as any haematologist will tell you, too much blood is a bad thing, it slows the circulation and can lead to thrombosis. To you as a manager committees will sometimes seem to have a life of their own, a malevolent alien life force sucking the energies of the organisation. However, if they are managed well by the chairman and participants they can move the process of management ahead speedily and effectively, but if they are managed badly they are one of the most frustrating wastes of time that you are likely to experience. I am saddened by the waste of time, talent and money reflected in getting together the people who attend those meetings; meetings in which multidisciplinary, well-behaved worthies sit about exchanging platitudes, bemoaning the difficulties, pledging cooperative working after in-depth reappraisals—where sharp-nosed chairladies call everyone by their Christian names and make a point of not leaving out the silent, dowdy lady from community care. And at the end of it there is frequently no conclusion, no plan of action that will be honoured, no righteous anger sent back up the line, no conspiratorial refusal to implement the unfunded and the unimplementable, no passionate plan to make happen what needs to happen, just a few well-rounded phrases in the minutes leading nowhere except to another committee meeting. It need not be like this!

You will, of course, have your own views about committees, but while the pressure sores of 8 years on committees remain painful and unhealed, I hope I am allowed some observations.

Any committee
Make sure you have set aside time from your clinical or other work so that you arrive promptly and can stay until the end. Clinicians have a very bad reputation for arriving late in their white coats looking smug and leaving early as if to see patients, but probably because they are bored. Always, always read the paperwork before the meeting, and if it did not reach you at least 24 hours before the meeting remonstrate at the meeting itself.

If there is an item on the agenda which is important to you and for which you need support try to talk to potential supporters and potential opponents before the meeting rather than expect to win them over during the meeting. Similarly if the item is important sit where the chairman can see you. If important decisions are made annotate your agenda papers with what was said and make sure that the minutes, when they subsequently emerge, accurately reflect what was agreed at the meeting.

If you are minded to set up a committee
Consider whether it is to achieve a defined purpose. If so, consider calling it a working party, give it a written remit and a timetable.

An unsatisfactory reason for setting up a committee is merely to allow colleagues to meet for a chat about mutually interesting issues. Even less acceptable are meetings to appease complaints about exclusion from the decision-making process by establishing a toothless talking shop.

If the committee is for the purpose of conducting necessary routine business (the usual reasons for having a committee)
It is important to know to whom it reports, whether it has an executive function and who sets the agenda. If you can not answer these questions then perhaps the committee should not exist, and you should consider whether some other less formal grouping will fulfil the task that you have in mind.

If you have been made chairman of a committee
If the committee meets regularly try to arrange for it to meet at intervals which can be calculated monthly or quarterly and at the same time and day of the week. A meeting with constantly changing times may seem a good idea in that no small group of members are particularly put out by having to change their timetables, but it invariably leads to confusion and is usually deemed unsatisfactory and scrapped.

When considering timing in the day, clinicians tend to find a 5 o'clock meeting or later the most convenient if it is to be a 1- or 2-hour meeting, but major meetings which will last at least 3 hours should be timetabled as a half-day. Some like breakfast meetings, "power breakfasts", though personally I think they are a sin for they encapsulate all the failures of the machismo management culture, viz:

- Failure to plan working timetables effectively.
- I can get up earlier than you!
- Failure to respect the private lives of contributors.

They are also gastronomically a disaster.

It has been noted that the length of committee meetings is proportional to the weight of the chairman. Thinner chairmen become hypoglycaemic and restive more quickly.

3.3.1 The conduct of committees

Remember that committees subserve several different functions.

(1) Information transmission.

(2) Commenting on and potentially altering proposed decisions.

(3) A truly open-ended debate on an issue with the purpose of formulating policy.

When managing the agenda of a meeting it is important that you are clear into which category each item will fall. Agendas can be usefully divided into items "for information", "for decision", or "for discussion". Where there is this clear division firm chairmanship is needed to ensure the players keep to it. There is a lot of Brownian movement in committees, grumbling and rumbling, toing and froing, and this tends to amplify itself such that all committees have an in built tendency to chaos. The more democratic and openly run they are the worse the risk. The danger in this is that the committee may fail to make decisions and those decisions are then merely made on another day by a smaller group.

There is a theoretical ideal composition for a committee, the character of whose different members so complement one another that the committee works perfectly. Psychologists love to appraise and analyse top teams (ideally for a fee) to see that there is the right mix of initiators, finishers, lateral thinkers, healers, etc. In the real world one does not, of course, have the luxury to pick the perfect mix, which anyway may not be as important as theorists assert; indeed one of the most functionally effective committees I have ever been on was assessed by professional psychologists to be, in theory, totally dysfunctional.

3.3.2 Are committees effective?

It would be nice to think that they are and it is a fact of life to discover that often they are not, but that should not dismay you. The alternatives after all are likely to be less palatable stop-off points on the continuum between dictatorship and mob rule. Committees are after all just part of the management process in which team members come together. Teams do not necessarily work well. The Cranfield Executive Development Survey of the dynamics of management groups in Britain and other European countries found that:

● 40% of general managers felt negative about the senior bosses.

40

- 58% of chairs, chief executive officers and managing directors felt uncomfortable about the effectiveness of the senior team and the performance of its members.
- 51% of chief executive officers, managing directors and general managers feel there are important and sensitive issues at top level which remain unaddressed.
- 63% of senior management recognise there are substantial hindrances to achieving objectives in the senior team.[7]

3.3.3 Ploys

You should be aware of a number of ploys that (other) people use in committees to get their own way:

(1) *Bludgeoning.* This is probably the simplest manoeuvre, it simply involves monopolising the conversation or the agenda until you get your own way, or refusing to support other people until they support you. This tends to be a surgeon's ploy; surgeons lust after action (often for its own sake) while physicians, happy in the cosy inglenooks of the intellect, prefer a quiet debate.

(2) *Any Other Business.* The item is slipped in at the end of the meeting under "Any Other Business" when the members are tired and some have left. Items for "Any Other Business" should therefore be declared at the beginning of the meeting.

(3) *The Tabled Paper.* This is where the paper presenting your argument is slipped onto the table during the meeting and other members of the committee have neither the time to read the paper nor the opportunity to check the facts. Tabled papers should not be allowed.

(4) *Await the absence of opponents.*

(5) *The Trojan Horse Manoeuvre.* This involves embedding the subject of your choice into some other non-contentious issue, either in the agenda papers or in the debate.

(6) *The Go-between Manoeuvre.* This is a variant of the Trojan horse manoeuvre and involves using a biddable and acceptable messenger to achieve your ends rather than putting it up yourself when people may be sensitised to you or your message.

(7) *Misrepresentation* of what the committee actually decided. Although this sounds like straightforward dishonesty it is, I suspect, more often simply that you hear what you wish to hear. Always check the minutes of the last meeting.

3.4 Time management

3.4.1 Controlling stress in the job

Taking on a management role while continuing as a clinician is a recipe for stress. This needs to be realised at the outset and steps taken to control it. Caplan's study of stress in GPs, hospital consultants, and hospital managers showed depression in 27%, 19%, and 6% respectively,[8] although depression need not of course be just a response to stress. A more recent study from Sheffield has, by contrast, shown that one in three NHS managers are suffering from stress, an approximately similar figure to doctors and nurses.[9] What is not yet known is what surplus stress or depression levels, if any, are experienced by clinicians who are also managers. Are natural copers selected for the job or do the conflicts and the workload inherent in the double job lead to stress symptoms? Or does having your hand on the reins protect from stress. From personal observations I have no doubt that "burn-out" can occur in clinician managers because of the insoluble frustrations of the job, just as it can in oncologists. Whether the stresses of clinical and management work done in parallel are synergistic needs to be explored. A study performed for the Association of Surgeons of Great Britain and Ireland[10] explored conflicts between administrative, clinical and personal life. There was a response from 305 of 975 Fellows. Seventy per cent described a conflict between administrative work and personal life during the previous 3 weeks, with 78% being resolved in favour of the administrative demand. Seventy-one per cent also reported conflicts between clinical and administrative work during the previous 3 weeks, with 49% being resolved in favour of the administrative demands. Worryingly 68% believed their work with patients had suffered at least once during the previous month because of stress.

What is clear is that the management of time is central to the management of stress, and that a little thought invested in planning time management at the outset of your appointment will pay dividends later. Management of the flow of information is also critical, though perhaps less easy to assess than problems with time management.

3.4.2 Time management

It is not natural for people to admit that they waste a good deal of their time at work, particularly when they see themselves as overworked, but bear in mind the Bareto 80/20 principle. Bareto was a nineteenth-century economist who noted that, for example, 20% of the workforce does 80% of the work, 20% of a document contains 80% of the useful information and so on. It must be assumed that your work potentially displays the same split and in arranging to manage time you want to get rid of as much of the 80% non-productive work as is possible. If you do not manage this you may find yourself with an uncontrolled workload punishing your family or yourself to the point when new and even more damaging stresses are introduced into your life. To cope with all this you need some strategies and the strength of purpose to observe them.

Firstly you need a *personal job plan*, a personal declaration of intent about how you plan to lead your life as a manager. This need not be public, it can be in your head, although if it is shared with your domestic partner it will be less easy to deny later that these were your objectives. For example:

> I am the clinical director for acute medical directorates. In addition to this I will take an interest in things to do with emergency medicine, primary care and elderly care. I am not personally interested in computing, New Deal or Calman, so I will avoid or delegate these. I will have breakfast with my children every day and will accept evening obligations on only two days a week. I will arrange events to allow me to visit the gym on Tuesdays and Thursdays at 6.00 pm etc.

A bit short but the right flavour. Having done that now some specific strategic directions:

Strategy one—A hard re-look at the timetable.
Have you yet scheduled one or more half-days when you are in your office? You need to do that and ensure that your secretary (now that you are a manager you will be calling him or her a PA!) knows that this is the only time to arrange for people to see you. Have you scheduled a regular team meeting and/or a walkabout session? All these should count as managerial "fixed sessions" in addition to any predictable committee work.

Strategy two—Dealing with the mail
There are many ways to solve this problem; for example get your PA to sort the mail into four separate heaps. Firstly, the clinical mail;

43

secondly, managerial material needing letters; thirdly, managerial documents needing reading and, fourthly, (usually the largest pile) material that can be thrown into the bin, for example invitations to seminars, the third blurred photocopy of the latest executive circular, advertising material, etc. Additionally you will need a carefully garnered pile of papers relating to impending committees. These should be clearly labelled, because everything nowadays is printed in Times New Roman typeface on "Word" and looks identical. Ideally it should be presented in a separate file containing the agenda, the minutes of the last meeting, etc.

Try not to leave in the evening before you have dealt with the mail and dictated on it where necessary. Just dumping it all into your briefcase to be dealt with at home is not the correct solution.

Although you should try not to handle any piece of mail any more than once, a "pending file" is useful. Things you think are probably unimportant but you are not entirely sure can be put in the file. When you check the file in 3 months time you will find most of it can go straight into the bin.

Treat e-mail in the same way as letters. If you set about reading your own e-mails on screen yourself (the average manager in the UK is said to receive 64 each day) you will be quickly bogged down in trivia and irrelevance, quite apart from suffering stress generated by the slovenly abuse of language that typifies e-mails.

Strategy three—Avoid interruptions

It is difficult to balance accessibility with the need to work effectively. Your clinical colleagues are the most difficult in this. Not only will they expect you to be able to fix things for them but they also want to tell you about it, at length—now! Very few people understand the stresses under which you work and few of them respect your time. Therefore leave your bleep/portable phone with someone outside when you are going into a meeting, have all the calls to your office passed through your secretary and, lastly, remain standing and close to the door when people "drop by" to see you without an appointment. These manoeuvres can, of course, be carried to extremes and it is irritating when telephoning others to be told that they are "in a meeting". The retort "what meeting is that?" or "is it a real meeting?" may elucidate whether your target is simply chatting to a colleague and can be disturbed. Remember, however, to treat others as you would wish them to treat you and that however urgently you feel you need to talk to the chief executive or the director of finance, he is as likely to be as frustrated by unstructured calls on his time as you are.

Strategy four—Avoid futile meetings

As a clinical or medical director you will be asked to many meetings simply from courtesy or because the arrangers wish to influence you. If the meeting is not part of your mainstream obligations or will not contribute to your personal objectives, do not accept. If you are in doubt as to whether this is the right course it is sometimes acceptable to ask if you could receive the minutes and agendas and come only if there are relevant items. You will have to learn to live with the anxiety that meetings you do not attend may decide something you do not agree with.

Inherent in all this is the ability to say "NO". The new consultant and the new medical manager tend to be flattered to be asked to do things and may not have a clear view of what saying "yes" will entail. So if asked *always* find out what saying "yes" lets you in for and then make a careful judgment in your own time rather than in the corridor. Saying "no" sounds selfish but it is not always so, it may be simply sensible.

Strategy five—Delegate

This does not mean ducking your responsibilities; it is a positive act that ensures that other team members have their skills used properly. Delegation can also be used as a good vehicle with which to "bring on" clinicians who have no current management responsibilities. Even the smallest task exposes them to the *realpolitik* of making the system work. It is sensible though, when delegating in this way, to outline the task, though not necessarily the process, and to give a timetable in writing. Remember not to delegate work which should simply be eliminated.

There is a useful management aphorism about prioritisation; "Do it, delegate it or discard it".

Strategy six—Manage the flow of information

As doctors we have well-structured ways for handling information; we read a selected, small group of journals and we know how we can retrieve that information via computer searches on Medline or by way of our personal filing system. We have books whose authors largely agree on how best to deal with any particular clinical problem. We go to meetings where the advice we receive is largely

45

consensual and probably has some scientific validity. It then comes as a rude shock to the new manager to be quickly buried by an avalanche of unstructured information.

At first it is impossible to determine what is necessary, what is useful, what might be useful in the future and indeed to determine which of all this stuff is true; what is a try on, what is propaganda and where is the kernel of this overripe information fruit that reports a policy which is real and will be acted upon. The information is untidily presented, heaps of verbose expensively printed reports vie for your attention with binders full of undigested data, beguilingly glossy free magazines, e-mails, faxes and photocopies slipped under the door by the invisible bumph fairy. The fruit of the information tree has an exceptionally low nutritional value even for a manager hungry to find out what it is that keeps this new world spinning. It is difficult to know what to file, what to open, what to read even, so the rookie manager needs quickly to learn the skills of skim reading, prioritisation and, most importantly, of throwing paper away. Be very wary of just putting things to one side or of filing them unread, for that only encourages an accusatory and depressing burden of information that will never be assimilable. A survey by Reuters found that half of 1300 managers questioned were suffering from a degree of information overload which, far from making their tasks easier as was intended, was actually leading to less ability to make a decision and to more stress.[11] The information overload does this simply because we are not able to assimilate the torrent of information and yet we feel we ought to for within the unassimilated information there might be the nugget that negates what we are about to decide. The urgency culture of the mobile phone and the e-mail implies that everything is genuinely important and can make the whole thing even more stressful. As this is a pandemic disease which society currently shows no desire to alleviate there is little the individual can do, but there is a lot to be said for *not* having a mobile phone, *not* having e-mail and leaving the answerphone switched off most of the time! Managerial matters are rarely that urgent and often benefit from composing in an in-tray for a while or waiting to be aired at the next scheduled committee meeting.

Strategy seven—Do all of this in the right environment
A good PA/secretary, an effective filing system, and a clear desk are essentials. Two to three comfortable chairs around a low table where you can have discussions are very helpful. You might even

explore the Feng Shui approach. Feng Shui is the ancient Chinese art of correct placement; if things in your environment are placed appropriately your life will be happier, easier, and more successful. However, given the limitations of Health Service space and budget your options for amending your environment with mirrors, large plants and wind chimes are likely to be seriously curtailed, so you may have to live with your chi running incorrectly through your space. The best you can do is avoid the omnipresent pressures of heaps of unresolved paperwork surrounding you on every flat surface. An empty desk is, indeed, a happy desk. I expect someone has said "show me a cluttered office and I will show you a cluttered mind"—I hope not!

3.5 Managing a budget

I didn't relish writing this section on the management of a budget. I am no exception in this; it is the management area that clinicians seem to like least. So I shared the problem with my undergraduate son when he was home for the weekend—"Managing a budget . . . what's the problem? You get given an amount of money and you just have to make it last." Ah! If only it were that simple, but therein lies the answer to the clinician's difficulty.

3.5.1 Problems about budget holding

The undergraduate, apart from a need to keep his food intake above starvation level, and to buy the occasional round, is the master of all the elements of his budget. Not so the clinician in management. He is probably aware that the evolving NHS has created the concept of the clinician in management almost solely as an attempt to control clinical budgets; he may agree with the concept; he may understand intellectually and emotionally that money is real and budgets are finite, but he personally spends only a tiny part of the budget and most of the expenditure within his directorate is historically based, inescapable, or driven by factors outside his control. The clinical manager's scepticism about the virtues of budget holding will be further fuelled by the fact that he is unlikely to have encountered a part of the NHS in which poor budgetary performance has led to closure or firings. By contrast, he will be familiar with the time-honoured response of overspending budget holders being rewarded with an increase in budget, while the under-spender is penalised by a reduction in next year's allocation. None of this is really a recipe for enthusiastic budget holding by clinicians. In addition, the clinical manager may find the paperwork daunting unless it is properly presented and he has been educated to understand it. So what should the clinical manager understand?

(1) The types of budgets that exist in an NHS unit.
(2) How data is commonly presented to the budget-holding medical manager.
(3) How the budget is set.
(4) The sort of options that clinical directors have to control budgets and expenditure.

3.5.2 Types of budget

It is important to identify the two types of accounting activity that trusts and other NHS organisations undertake:

(1) *Financial accounting* sometimes called stewardship accounting. This is the accounting to the people who provide the money to show that it has been properly used. Such accounting is usually annual and historical. NHS trusts are accountable to the NHS executive. Their accounting will include items of income and expenditure, reviews of their assets, their use of capital, and so on. It is outside the scope of this chapter.

(2) *Management accounting.* This is the kind of accounting that the medical manager will deal with and she should not be sceptical about the need for it. It is simply a management tool that involves the setting of budgets and the production of regular, useful accounts, usually on a monthly basis, that look back at expenditure and look forward to determine whether expenditure will match income. They seem natural now, but in 1978 the Royal Commission on the NHS noted an almost complete absence of them. "Working for Patients" in 1989, whatever its other failings, did at least help to establish prudent accountancy practice as a mainstream feature of NHS management. Management accounting should underpin the running of any business because, quite simply, it helps the manager balance income with expenditure and may help her explore the areas which need attention. Lastly, of course, it provides the data which allows her to write a credible business plan.

There is another sort of accounting "cost accounting"; this is a specialised discipline allowing accurate costing of products in the commercial sector. It is not generally used within the NHS.

As a clinical director you discover that there are two parts to the management accounting in relation to your service. One is the *central budget* which describes the core function of the organisation, including obvious things like facilities, catering, rates, electricity, and also less obvious items like reserves and capital charges. The other is your *directorate budget*, which concerns expenditure by your team in your directorate. In assessing costs, these two budgets must be reconciled.

The central budget is always larger than clinical directors think it ought to be, but defining it is a complex area left to the finance department. If, however, you are involved in price setting for contracts you will need to know the details of those central costs. You are, of course, allowed to be critical if they seem to be profligate.

Directorate budgets

Managing your own directorate budget will require you to slot into a budget cycle of *setting, reporting, reviewing,* and then the familiar biological feedback cycle that also applies to audit, whereby the reviewing informs the next cycle of *setting* and so on.

Budget setting

This is done by the chief executive and/or the director of finance, but must involve you, your business manager and finance manager, otherwise we fall into the old NHS trap of divorcing budget planning from operational management. Traditional budget setting occurs in advance of the financial year and is supposed to be concluded by March, although it may be difficult to achieve this if there are delays in concluding contracts, getting allocations from the NHS Executive and so on.

The budget as set is usually historical with extra cash allocated for medical advances, inflation, etc., together with additional contractual work. From this is subtracted any efficiency savings expected of you, or any fraction of an overall income loss that the trust is experiencing which is to be passed on to your directorate. Last year's overspend or underspend may also be reflected in this year's budget. All of that is the "top down" element.

49

The "bottom up" part of the process is what your clinical directorate brings to the debate. This is rarely part of the negotiation about the budget to be set, but is more often part of the process of looking to see how genuine cost pressures which your directorate will experience can be met from within your budget. Examples of such cost pressures might include the implementation of Calman training reforms, or the separation of male wards from female wards. Also to be taken into account are initiatives arising from your own directorate business plan which you will want to put into your calculations. Remember when doing that that satisfying demands for information, for extra teaching, for audit, for quality improvements will often have a price tag attached: "Yes, we'll happily do that but it will cost £xx in the next financial year". These figures also need to go into the brew. There is an element of negotiation between you and the director of finance in all this, but the director's room for manoeuvre will probably be very limited and your increased costs are unlikely to be reflected in extra income for the trust. At the end of this process you would, in traditional terms, be set a fixed budget, or possibly a partly flexible budget; the flexible element reflects unpredictable workloads beyond your control but only if this extra activity will be funded.

You will also at this point need to be clear what the plans are for the management of over- or underspends during the coming year, particularly whether you have an option to use revenue underspends on capital equipment and, lastly, what level of expenditure you are personally authorised to commit. The rules relating to the clinical director's power personally to approve expenditure differ from one organisation to another, but each will have "standing financial instructions" which you ought to read (very boring but very important!), especially in relation to the upper limits of spending which the clinical director is allowed.

The 1998 reforms will make the budget setting process more difficult. Expenditure control will remain as important as ever, but the "abolition" of the internal market will make the ability to manage income potentially more difficult because income will be more fixed than it was in the days of the "internal market" and less likely to be responsive to workload.

When the budget is finally set you *must* be clear what elements of the budget can be controlled and what can realistically be achieved. This is where your clinical knowledge is crucial and where everybody must be clear about what is controllable and what is not. The finance director and the chief executive also need to be clear about this. It does not do the organisation a favour to start the year with unreasonable or overoptimistic budgetary expectations, yet one sees it over and over again, leading to crises of cancellation and media interest each winter, usually echoed by government ministers blaming the service for inept management.

Cost improvement programmes

"Cost improvement" means "cost reduction", you can't *improve* on a cost but *improvement* sounds good so it's there to blunt the sting. So abjectly submissive to these "weasel words"[12] have we become that I missed this one until none other than John Pelly our Director of Finance pointed out how misleading the term is. Unfortunately we're stuck with it.

If big chunks are to be taken out of the budget, either for an explicit cost improvement programme or because of a previous unresolved overspend, the mechanics of those savings should be explicit and agreed at the outset and communicated to all the team. There is nothing more depressing and unachievable for a clinical director than to be told part way through the year that the expected out-turn needs to be reduced by a large amount.

Specific cost improvement programmes must be accurately costed, their progress monitored and, in general, they should be achieved without a reduction in workload. Even if cost pressures are discounted, it becomes increasingly difficult year on year to achieve significant cost improvements once the obvious targets such as overstaffing, length of stay and day surgery rates have been addressed. Simply *not* doing things is the next option. For example, limiting the number of investigations or procedures for a disease or simplifying drug therapy. If this is to be done without reducing the quantity of care provided, it can only be informed by properly researched evidence-based medicine (EBM) protocols, few of which are in existence. There is of course a snag in this that for every cost saving EBM protocol, there may be an equal number of cost-increasing protocols. The merging of clinical departments between hospitals is another option, but this rarely produces the large savings needed, even though such savings will usually have been adduced as the reason for a merger.

Budget reporting

The budget, once set, will need to be reported on monthly. If you, the clinical director, are going to be able to respond usefully to those reports, they will need to be:

- accurate
- timely
- understandable
- relevant
- consistent
- agreed.

There is no virtue in the report containing "fixed costs" such as rent and rates and capital charges, because the clinical director cannot influence these. The actual report will need to show so-called "semi-fixed" costs, such as:

- nursing salaries
- consultant salaries
- administrative and clerical salaries

  and "variable" costs such as:

- theatre charges
- cross-charges for meals and portering
- drugs
- pathology tests
- theatre disposables.

It will need clearly to identify agency and locum staff costs as these tend to be a source of nasty surprises.

The lines are subdivided into columns: the annual budget, sometimes called the plan, this month's budget, this month's actual spend, variance from the plan and some sort of full-year projection with the variance to show how your budget is likely to end the year. Be familiar with the notations used, especially where it signifies an overspend. Figures in brackets may signify a gain or underspend as they do in Figure 3.1 but in other organisations they may signify the opposite! To make managerial sense of these figures, you will also need to see some basic activity and staffing date such as finished consultant episodes, admissions and waiting lists, again presented as predicted and actual figures. Lastly it is helpful to know what your staff levels are in relation to establishment. It is sometimes possible to include all this data for a directorate on a single sheet of paper.

GUY'S AND St. THOMAS' NHS HOSPITAL TRUST 1998/99

FINANCIAL PERFORMANCE REPORT FOR THE PERIOD: APRIL TO JULY

VASCULAR SURGERY

99 S-03-831

WTE BUDGET	WTE ACTUAL	JULY BUDGET £	JULY SPEND £	JULY VARIANCE £			ANNUAL BUDGE £	TO DATE BUDGET £	TO DATE SPEND £	VARIANCE TO DATE £
						MEDICAL STAFF				
1.36	1.36	9065	8583	(482)	MC210	CONSULTANT	108769	36234	34402	(1832)
	1.00	3830	3552	(278)	MC21M	CONSULTANT MEDICAL SCHOOL	45963	15321	14984	(337)
2.00		0	1452	1452	MN410	SENIOR REGISTRAR	0	0	16851	16851
		8257	916	(8257)	MN250	SPEC REGISTRAR	99096	33000	12222	(20778)
		0	0	916	MN25M	SPR REGISTRAR	0	0	2748	2748
1.00	1.00	3316	11969	8653	MN210	SENIOR HOUSE OFFICER	39811	13254	11969	(1285)
3.00	3.00	6824	6463	(361)	MN110	HOUSE OFFICER	81890	27250	26064	(1186)
1.00	1.00	0	13924	13924	MN25L	SPR REGISTRAR LOCUM	0	0	13924	13924
0.66		2156	0	(2156)	MN31L	REGISTRAR LOCUM	25891	8619	0	(8619)
		888	0	(888)	ZADH0	ADDITIONAL DUTY HOURS	10652	3551	931	(2621)
8.02	7.36	34336	46859	12523		TOTAL MEDICAL STAFF	412072	137229	134095	(3134)
						NURSING STAFF				
1.00	1.00	2131	2127	(4)	NX010	SNR NURSE PRACTITIONER	25568	8523	8509	(14)
1.00	1.00	2131	2127	(4)		TOTAL NURSING STAFF	25568	8523	8509	(14)
						ADMIN & CLERICAL				
1.00	1.00	1733	1706	(27)	CR31S	MEDICAL SECRETARY 4	20789	6930	6823	(107)
2.00		2941	(1704)	(4645)	C000M	ADMIN & CLERICAL MEDICAL SCH	35298	11766	13787	2021
		545	(1694)	(2239)	C000A	ADMIN & CLERICAL STAFF AGENCY	6550	2183	9327	7144
3.00	1.00	5219	(1692)	(6911)		TOTAL ADMIN & CLERICAL	62637	20879	29937	9058

Figure 3.1 An example of a financial performance report. This is a monthly report for the clinical director of surgery and concerns the vascular surgical unit. The costs of theatre time, outpatients and the use of the team's own beds are not included in this budget. The clinical director will see them on the report for the whole directorate.

GUY'S AND St. THOMAS' NHS HOSPITAL TRUST 1998/99
FINANCIAL PERFORMANCE REPORT FOR THE PERIOD: APRIL TO JULY
VASCULAR SURGERY
99 S-03-831

WTE BUDGET	WTE ACTUAL	JULY BUDGET £	JULY SPEND £	JULY VARIANCE £	Code	Description	ANNUAL BUDGET £	TO DATE BUDGET £	TO DATE SPEND £	VARIANCE TO DATE £
						NON PAY				
		0	0	0	2B000	STAFF UNIFORMS	10	3	0	(3)
		6656	5355	(1301)	2D00E	Drugs Expend Cross Charge	79880	26627	28128	1501
		6914	5524	(1390)	2DHE1	Blood Products Exp Cross Charge	82967	27656	24380	(3276)
		12	0	(12)	2F000	MEDICAL & SURGICAL EQUIPMENT	150	50	0	(50)
		5590	0	(5590)	2G000	PATIENTS APPLIANCES	67080	22360	9235	(13125)
		0	2016	2016	2GSA0	surgical appliances	0	0	5191	5191
		7	0	(7)	2P000	ELECTRICAL APPLIANCES	90	30	0	(30)
		6	0	(6)	2W000	RESUS PRINTING & STATIONERY	73	24	12	(12)
		28	0	(28)	2WA00	COMPUTER HARDWARE	346	115	1463	1348
		186	0	(186)	2WH00	STATIONERY	2231	744	17	(727)
		99	0	(99)	3DA00	ADVERTING COSTS	1183	395	250	(395)
		20	0	(20)	3DE01	TRAINING & ED COURSE FEES	230	77	0	173
		0	(403)	(403)	3DR00	REMOVAL EXPENSES	0	0	0	0
		152	0	(152)	3DT00	TRAVEL & SUBSISTENCE	1834	611	385	(226)
		7	0	(7)	3DT01	EXCESS TRAVEL EXPENSES	90	30	22	(8)
		89	515	426	3X00M	MED PHOTO-MED SCH RECHARGE	1072	357	715	358
		2	0	(2)	3X00P	PHOTOCOPYING - MED SCH RECHARGE	31	10	0	(10)
		17	0	(17)	3XM9M	MED/SCH ULTRASONIC ANGIOLOGY	204	68	0	(68)

Figure 3.1 contd

Code	Description							
9AM80	PATIENTS TRANSPORT RECHARGE	743	980	237	8909	2970	3094	124
9B000	MINI CAB/TAXI RECHARGES	2	0	(2)	24	8	0	(8)
9BEDS	USE OF BEDS CROSS CHARGE	0	350	350	0	0	490	490
9CC01	TELEPHONE RECHARGES	56	0	(56)	668	223	566	343
9EITU	ITU Recharges inwards	21327	18406	(2921)	255928	85309	36826	(48483)
9ENUC	EXP NUCLEAR MEDICINE RECHARGES	679	281	(398)	8141	2714	1123	(1591)
9EPCH	EXP CHEM PATH TESTS	3245	4242	997	38957	12985	13853	868
9EPHA	EXP HAEMATOLOGY TESTS	3662	4826	1164	43940	14647	16723	2076
9EPHI	EXP HISTOPATHOLOGY TESTS	9717	16494	6777	116603	38868	50791	11923
9EPIM	EXP IMMUNOLOGY TESTS	186	560	374	2236	745	1506	761
9EPMI	EXP MICROBIOLOGY TESTS	3916	4108	192	46994	15665	15546	(119)
9EPVI	EXP VIROLOGY TESTS	262	600	338	3154	1051	1716	665
9ERAD	EXP RADIOLOGY INTERNAL RECHARG	28120	27664	(456)	337441	112480	115765	3285
9HOSP	CATERING HOSPITALITY RECHARGE	0	0	0	0	0	10	10
9PC00	IT TRAINING RECHARGES	10	0	(10)	120	40	0	(40)
9PC04	IT INSTALLATIONS/LICENCES RECH	0	0	0	0	0	100	100
9PH00	PHOTOCOPYING RECHARGE	0	0	0	0	0	5	5
9****	TOTAL INTERNAL RECHARGES	71925	78511	6586	863115	287705	258114	(29591)
	TOTAL NON PAY SPEND	91710	91517	(193)	1100586	366862	327912	(38950)
	TOTAL THIS REPORT	133396	138812	5416	1600863	533493	500453	(33040)

12.02   9.36

Figure 3.1 *contd*

55

The trust as a whole will have similar but larger sheets covering all of its business, divided up by its separate component services.

You can try to use all this information to yield a price per procedure, or a cost per case. In theory this will allow you comparison between your patients and those of other services or directorates, or even other hospitals, but the variability in case mix, the crudeness of cost allocations and the primitiveness of NHS information technology, makes the figures largely meaningless. The drive to produce these figures was once an inherent need of the internal market and is still pursued for its own sake. Sadly, though, the NHS has never realised that information is not a free good, nor to my knowledge has there ever been a cost–benefit analysis of whether *detailed* knowledge of cost can be shown to alter the total cost of healthcare or to improve it within the NHS. In the USA and in the UK private sector, where activity is funded on a cost-per-case basis, such costing activities are inescapable. Costing as an obsession is however here to stay and the case mix issue is being addressed; thus you may need to be familiar with the concept of DRGs (diagnosis-related groups). There are several hundred of these and, in theory, each can be separately costed, but they are crude. In the UK the tendency has been to use HRGs (healthcare resource groups), which are more sophisticated as they combine diagnosis, secondary diagnoses and procedures. It may be possible to make them more accurate by adding severity scores. Eventually, may be, meaningful costings and perhaps even outcome analyses will be available.

It is not your job as medical manager to construct these equations, but you do need to try to ensure that these complicated financial activities do not drift too far away from clinical reality. As far as your own budget sheet is concerned the structure and the figures need to be devised between your business manager and the finance directorate. You do need to know not only the director of finance in your organisation, but also the person responsible for monitoring and constructing your budget. In big hospitals with big finance departments this may be difficult but it is important for there to be an identifiable person. Some would say that that person should be *managerially* accountable to you while *professionally* accountable to the director of finance. I am not convinced that accountability to you the clinical director is crucial, but it is important that a named person is responsible for the accuracy of your budget sheets.

Reviewing and controlling expenditure in a clinical directorate

So here you are at your monthly review meeting, cup of coffee in hand, budget statement in front of you and your team eager to discuss what is needed.

An example of the sort of budget statement which you might have is shown in Figure 3.1.

It is month 4 (that's finance speak for July), things are going well. There are some "year to date expenditures" which are less than planned. Can you spend the surplus? Probably not! Look very closely to see why this unusual state of affairs has obtained. There is a small overall underspend on medical staff but a big overspend on medical staff this month which you need to sort out because if it continues through the year it may wreck your budget. Staff underspends due to unfilled vacancies are OK, unless the staff agency bill simply hasn't been paid yet. Lower than expected use of consumables is OK, but only if it accurately reflects what has already been bought or committed which is very unusual. Non-pay expenditure is always difficult to track accurately because you need to measure expenditure commitments as well as actual expenditure. It is quite common for things to look good mid-year, only to slip as the year goes on. In the example shown here you can see that the ITU cross-charging budget is underspent, or is it? Again you will need to know if this truly represents a change in practice leading to less demand for ITU beds or is it just the vagaries of the billing process or is it a temporarily low throughput. Also note on this budget sheet how financially trivial are many of the lines (where you might be tempted to act) and that there are big sums in some lines such as blood products and radiology where changed clinical practice might produce real savings if you need them.

In the more common scenario, either things are looking unsatisfactory right now, or your year-end projections are unsatisfactory. What should you do? First check the data to find out why things are off plan. If there is a good clinical reason, for instance to do with volume of admissions, you will need to discuss this promptly with the chief executive and/or director of finance to agree a way for handling the problem. Simply stopping elective admissions towards year-end is a primitive and unsatisfactory response and only saves significant quantities of money if beds are closed and staff levels reduced. If the problem is not admissions, the causes of an overspend are sometimes due to clinical behaviour, quirky changes in bed occupancy or drug use for instance. More often the problem is agency staff or locum use, or overtime. The difficulty with all overspends on staff (who are likely to account for 70% of your budget) is the lag time in getting control of expenditure, either by reducing or increasing numbers or doing away with the need for agencies and locum staff. This is caused by the cost and cumbersomeness of personnel processes. You need, therefore, to keep ahead of the game and to make sure that the agreed and funded establishment is realistic and sufficient to cover leave, etc.

Changing team behaviour at short notice is difficult, often impossible, and so, boring and nannyish as it may seem to clinicians, regular briefings about the state of the budget and exhortations to prudence are as important as any specific measures.

If things are uncorrectably overspent, then there may be grounds for the use of contingency funds. How best this should be arranged is debatable. Personally we favour a situation whereby the director of finance holds the contingency reserves and doles them out meanly, grudgingly and only after the most persuasive arguments are put to him.

Capital management
Even quite small directorates will have capital projects, even if they are only for the replacement of equipment. The processes by which trusts obtain capital is complex and outside the scope of this chapter, nevertheless it is important to realise that a finite amount of capital is available to a trust. This will comprise "minor block capital" for the routine replacement of equipment etc., and may also contain funding for larger capital items. Within a trust bids for capital will always exceed the amount available and all medical managers will need to understand the local process and timetable for bidding for capital. However that process is to be undertaken, a proven business case may need to be made for anything large or new, and that business case may need to include an option appraisal—one of the options always being that no capital is made available. Details of the business planning process are included in the next section.

Conclusion
There is nothing scary about holding a budget if the process is managed competently by all parties and if you have a good working

relationship with your department of finance. What is scary is an inappropriately set budget which leaves you with an impossible target, or incorrect or incomplete data which leaves you uncertain as to what is actually happening.

3.6 Business planning

> I keep six honest serving men,
> they taught me all I knew;
> Their names are What and Why and When
> And How and Where and Who.
> (RUDYARD KIPLING, The Elephant's Child)

No book on management is complete without a section on business planning and no business is complete without planning, yet "business planning" as an activity is the *bête noire* of managers and for many clinicians it is the managerial straitjacket formalised into print. By contrast, clinical trainees looking towards an impending interview may see it as the one bit of the managerial mystique which they need to understand.

What does business planning mean? Simply it implies not just thought, research and debate about the future of the business but, crucially, the ability to distil the conclusions into a single document to which the business should work in the succeeding year or longer.

For the medical manager we can usefully divide business planning into three groups of activities:

(1) The corporate plan.
(2) The directorate plan.
(3) The business plan for a specific project.

3.6.1 The corporate plan

The corporate plan is the all-embracing plan that trusts are required to produce for the NHS executive each year. It must incorporate the plans of all the individual directorates, reflect purchasers' intentions, respond to general changes in the NHS and include a response to major budget changes. Corporate plans are not produced in one sweep but evolve slowly over a year or more. The outlines that will eventually form the final business plan are the agendas for negotiations with purchasers, other health authorities and the NHS Executive. As well as setting the corporate priorities they are the starting point for directorate business plans. During the evolution of the corporate business plan there may be as many as a dozen timetabled review points when, for example, purchasers' intentions are circulated, prices decided, formal reviews of directorate plans undertaken and, finally, the point when the business plan is signed off by the NHS Executive. Details of such a process are outside the scope of this book, they are all very time consuming and not for the fainthearted. The average medical manager needs to know about the simpler but similarly structured construction of a directorate plan and to help achieve these the manager's trust should circulate explicit guidelines.

3.6.2 The directorate plan

The making of a directorate's business plan is not an esoteric activity. It is a simple exercise in common sense. The more down to earth it is the more credible it will be. The pulling together of the written business plan requires first that you do your planning properly; you are not simply reacting to a checklist sent down from the chief executive's office—or you shouldn't be. You should nevertheless have the list of corporate objectives in your hand when you start your own planning process. This is the "top down" planning document. What you need to add is your "bottom up" planning insights. Top down and bottom up should meet harmoniously in your final document.

The planning process at its simplest requires you to answer some questions.

(a) For what length of time are we planning?
The time is usually 1 year, but with a 2- to 3-year horizon against which to make longer-term plans. Ten-year plans are not really worth making because they are usually overtaken by unpredictable events.

(b) What do we want to do?
This is the bottom up part. This can only be derived from a proper knowledge of the directorate's work. Is there some new skill the team wishes to deploy? Do they want to start an innovative type

of clinic? Do you want to swap from inpatient to day care? Do you wish to appoint an extra consultant and so on.

(c) What do others want us to do?
This is the top down bit which requires that you know the corporate strategy. This may be a major change of service, for example, transferring radiotherapy to another trust or a response to a national initiative such as setting a firm target for outpatient waiting times which you will be expected to meet regardless of where it might come in your own hierarchy of targets. Additionally you will need to review messages from purchasers about what they want, from GPs, from patients (if you know), and from other directorates. These last are not really top down plans, more "sideways across" plans, but that's not proper management speak!

(d) What's the probable budget?
It would be nice if that didn't appear so soon in the list, and in traditional business planning texts it doesn't, but within the Health Service it will invariably be a major issue so it should not be left out of the reckoning for too long. I have seen too many NHS trust corporate business planning documents full of fine words about the extra things that need to be done, followed with barely a blink by detailed sums of expected reductions in budget, sometimes frankly put, sometimes dressed up as "cash releasing efficiency savings" to make you feel better about it. Either way it may clip the wings of your grand plans early.

(e) How do we integrate the demands of (b),(c) and (d)?
How do we integrate the demands of others with our own and turn them into an *achievable and affordable* set of objectives? To answer this takes time and consultation, brainstorming sessions, discussion papers, and meetings. The solutions that you come up with need to be accepted by the bulk of the team within your directorate and their *ownership* of the final plan is crucial.

(f) What resources will we need?
You will in part have answered this when refining your options, but now is the time to be more explicit about:

● Finance and the sources of it.

- Staff—do we need more or less? Will they have different roles? Be of different grades? And if we are in need of new staff what are the recruitment plans?
- Beds.
- Theatres.
- Services from other directorates, etc.

(g) What will be the impact on other directorates?

Will our closing, expanding or moving of a service completely undermine the functions of another directorate? Will we need more X-rays or pathology tests. Have we costed them? Can the relevant directorate provide them and at the cost we expect? In dealing with this last issue you need to understand the stepwise progression that characterises the enlargement of many Health Service facilities. You can understand this most easily perhaps in relation to ordering tests. It may be that the pathology department's machines and the staff who look after them are not currently working to capacity. Extra tests can therefore be done at a small incremental cost. It may be however that your extra demands will require them to purchase a new machine and possibly even employ more staff. This can dramatically alter the cost of your proposals.

Most business plans undertaken by directorates have a habit of neglecting a large number of extra costs incurred by other directorates, simple things like extra meals and transport costs for patients.

Now you are just about in a position to write your business plan. First though get out last year's plan!

3.6.3 Writing the business plan

This is one person's job. Not necessarily the most senior in the directorate but someone who from the outset of the process has kept in his hands all the threads that must be drawn together to make the plan. This will mean getting hold of data, retaining the papers from purchasers, etc., keeping a record of internal decisions. The business plan itself has for some reason developed a standard format, but I don't see why you need to stick to that. For a start it traditionally begins with a "mission statement". Personally I have a serious allergy to these and I am not alone in that. They tend to state the obvious, which in itself does no harm and can act as a gate through which all business proposals must pass, but to a reader of any intelligence they are an irritation and may well discourage him from taking the remainder of the document seriously. For example, the following was proposed as an example of a medical directorate's mission statement.[13]

The Medical Directorate aims to provide high quality medical care in a cost efficient manner. It seeks to provide equal access to its services, will ensure the privacy and dignity of its patients, and will promote the wellbeing of its workforce. It will support research and education and seeks to gain a reputation for outstanding clinical practice.

This, the authors imply, will be memorable and positive and act as a "focus and inspiration for the Directorate". I would submit that the average professional doctor and nurse or other in the directorate reading that mission statement might reply "what the hell do you think we are already doing? Are you suggesting that we currently don't do these things?" The answer of course may be "Yes, we are suggesting you are not doing them", but there are subtler ways of doing it. I have heard the angry responses to mission statements so many times and constructive responses so rarely that one wonders why managers insist on continuing with this amateurish spin doctoring. The most effective criticism is a practical one. The problem with fine words and heroic sentiments (fuzz and bullshit) is that they rarely point to any obvious action plan, so let's hope you have, instead of a mission statement, a down to earth ten-line introduction to your business plan saying what you wish to achieve. This is the same sort of statement that you would put at the beginning of a paper that you submit to a journal. The rest of the plan is not particularly contentious and a typical business plan might go as follows:

(1) *Summary introduction.*
(2) *Current position in relation to*: Long-term strategy. Redefine it. Is it still appropriate? How do directorate and corporate plans link in and then add some guesswork about future changes that will affect the directorate, new technology, and so on.
(3) *Last year's business plan*: How did we do? (be honest). What went well, what went badly, what are the messages for this year?

(4) *A brief SWOT analysis in relation to the options which might be in your new plan.* (SWOT = Strengths, Weaknesses, Opportunities, Threats analysis). For example:

Strength—We have a large number of diabetic patients.

Weakness—We do not have a good ophthalmic service dealing with diabetic retinopathy.

Opportunity—We are about to appoint a new ophthalmologist. This could be one of his special interests.

Threats—We will need extra laser equipment for which we do not have provision in the budget. Additionally, the trust down the road has just bought this equipment for themselves.

(5) *The proposed tactical plan*: This identifies how you are going to get on with your core business more efficiently and with better quality, and it also looks at your tactics for any new developments which you might wish to establish, for example your diabetic retinopathy service. In writing that plan you need to identify *who* carries responsibility for achieving each tactical move, *what resources* will be needed, and *what the timetable is*. Remember to include plans for communicating intentions and for training in relation to any change. Lastly it's prudent to spell out contingency arrangements if slippage occurs in the implementation of the plan.

(6) *Proposals for assessment*: What are the end points you hope to achieve? How and when are you going to measure them? Who will be responsible for that? In what format will those measurements be delivered?

(7) *Data underpinning all of the above*: This is financial and activity data, etc., together with contextual papers such as purchasers' intentions, corporate budget, patients charter standards, and so on. Enough data should be in your plan for an independent assessor to make a judgment about the plan. This is no different from writing a scientific paper, where you must present the data to justify your conclusions. The data in this instance can most easily be presented as an appendix.

(8) *Presentation of the plan*. Most of the value in the business planning process is in having to undergo the discipline of arriving at the point when you can write the plan clarifying your direction. But you will of course also need to communicate the decisions, so you need a full-length business plan replete with data and appendices for people who will know what they are looking at. Even so, advice is that such a document should

not exceed 20 pages. You will need a shorter, more easily readable version for communicating your plans outside the directorate and crucially to each member of the team inside the directorate.

I have used as a model the annual business plan for a directorate, but for many clinical directors their most considered planning will be directed to a specific service improvement or training issue. This may seem much more important to them than the annual business plan. The planning processes should, however, be much the same but it needs to lead to a crisper document. Clinicians who come to you with a bright, innovative idea (in truth or in their imagination) often resent being asked to turn it into a business plan and present it to you formally. They may need to be offered expert managerial help in preparation of the document but a plan is needed.

Curiously some NHS Executive projects don't seem to be subject to the rigours of a proper business case analysis before being sent down the line for implementation. Where so called "cost neutral" but obviously costly projects are wished on to you it is important to make your own realistic business case assessment early on in the process. A classic case of the inadequately funded initiative to emerge recently is the Calman training scheme. I have seen two excellent, crisp business planning assessments of the implications of implementing the Calman proposals. The preamble listed the nitty-gritty of what the proposals required of the trust, then defined the strategy for dealing with those proposals, then put them in the context of other initiatives underway, analysed the resources needed and the changed practice that could be expected, and, lastly, identified the costs in detail. These came out at between £600 000 and one million pounds per trust. When undertaking this kind of "defensive" business planning, the process needs to be just as rigorous as when you are the initiator.

3.6.4 The other view

The other view of business planning is that it has become a sterile, cultural ritual in the world of management and that it not only wastes time and stultifies fluidity, but it rarely encourages real change. The changes which can evolve within a properly managed unit can do so without formal planning processes and indeed may happen more efficiently and more quickly. They may do this because a business plan tends to be budget driven and by its sheer ponderousness can crush many initiatives at birth.

The cynical and more practical criticism of business plans is that no one reads them and that that doesn't matter because what they outline rarely happens. (The possible causal relationship between these two events often eludes the complainant!)

In spite of this we really cannot claim to be managing an NHS if we do not sign up to an intellectually credible planning process. Without it the business of management runs a risk of being static or merely reactive and has no route by which to escape the bondage of short-term constraints. However, don't forget that any business plan, to be acceptable amongst sceptical clinicians, must be:

- relevant
- explicit
- achievable
- affordable
- measurable
- and most crucially, owned. In fact a good NHS business plan is the mechanism by which clinicians can be drawn into involvement in the planning process.

3.7 Managing for quality

Quality in business is the way to success and fortune.

The only business goal of substance is the pursuit of quality[14]

In the NHS it is an unregarded poor relation. If you ask NHS staff what they are doing to improve the quality of the service you are likely to be met by incomprehension, for it is too often assumed that everybody is doing their best and that any failures of quality are failures of funding.

3.7.1 What is quality?

Quality of medical care should properly be about clinical outcomes; in essence "was the patient's presenting problem made better or improved, with the minimum of harm along the way?" But outcomes are very difficult accurately to assess and it is more normal, as we shall see later, to look at the *process* of care rather than the clinical results of the care. High-quality *process* may indeed be a surrogate for quality of outcome, but the danger is that these are simply changes which improve the smoothness of the process. They appeal more to the politics of gesture and are more immediately comprehensible to patients, so they may attract more attention than those which genuinely influence the outcome. It will always be exceptionally difficult to assess the *quality* of a Health Service as a global attribute because quality is a product of so many things, often evanescent and only distantly related to the end product, health. How long you are in the waiting room prior to your first consultation about your diabetes is only remotely associated with how well you can see 10 years later because of diabetic retinopathy. Nevertheless, the assumption that nothing can be done to improve quality in the Health Service is clearly erroneous, but it is deep rooted and the first step must be to move it up the agenda.

It also needs to be remembered that there is more to "quality" in healthcare than the patients' experience of their treatment; there are also issues about access and equality which are as important as process and outcome.

3.7.2 The disregard of quality

In the Health Service the reasons why an obsession with quality is not high on the agenda might be summarised as follows:

- Improved quality does not impinge on the success of the business even though the competition between providers envisaged by "Working for Patients" reforms was intended to achieve this. As a business objective it has always taken third place to productivity and cost effectiveness.
- No one loses their job if quality is consistently poor.
- There is little consumer pressure to increase quality and what there is is directed to headline topics such as single-sex wards. What pressure there is is weak and often misdirected.
- The resources needed to improve quality are only rarely available and the exhortation that quality improvements do not imply the spending of money is perceived as false by those working in the service.
- In a conservative service familiar only with incremental change, the radical changes needed to improve quality may simply demand too much time and effort from staff to get started.

- There are no easily available comparators to show where quality is poor.
- Although many official *pronouncements* speak of the need to bend the service to the needs of its customers the patients, official *actions* are likely to show that the true customers being served are the taxpayers.

Thus, moves towards improved quality are occurring against the grain of the primary activities of the organisation, and the pressures to improve quality are normally simply a matter of professional pride to the workers in the Health Service, rather than the result of a concerted and managerial effort.

As if to confirm this, "quality" is usually relegated to a non-mainstream department run by nurses with little or no input from clinicians and other professional groups.

The cynic may slyly observe that a central government's demands for quality are often simply a pre-emptive defensive ploy to minimise the damage done by a concurrent exercise in productivity and cost reduction. That aside, there is still an enormous amount that the clinician manager could and should do to improve quality. However, in doing so the manager need not read the copious management texts that exist on the subject; these publications first sprang from a different world when American businesses were trying to work out why Japanese products were overtaking theirs. A few concepts are transferable, but all you really need to do is to make an honest appraisal of the altogether more complicated world of healthcare at your door, most of whose priorities have nothing to do with the world of commerce. Patients are emphatically not customers. As a friend of mine who has spent much of the last 30 years in and out of hospital once said:

> I only ask three things of the Health system. Professionalism, Compassion and Privacy.

> (J. PARKER, Personal Communication)

3.7.3 Traditional quality arrangements in the NHS

It has always been assumed that a quality service will be delivered by the professionals within the service as an automatic byproduct of the fact that they are professionals. This has led to individual professional groups taking responsibility for the quality of their own service. The doctors' professional performance is regulated by professionals groups, Royal Colleges, the General Medical Council (GMC) and informed by other initiatives such as the Confidential Enquiry into Post Operative Deaths (CEPOD). The internal track record is scrutinised through clinical audit. The nurses traditionally had Matron, that stickler for quality in dress standards and the details of nursing care. Physiotherapists, speech therapists, radiographers, medical physicists, etc. all have their quality assurance programmes. It is fashionable to assume that this process is archaic and unable to deliver quality. In fact, these internal professional processes have quietly catalysed progressive increments in the quality of care for generations. Recently one might have noted that the CEPOD was a joint initiative by the surgeons and the anaesthetists; that the improvements in nursing education and practice and the development of the nurse practitioner grade were orchestrated by nursing organisations. The whole exercise of audit and Evidence Based Medicine (EBM) is not a product of the government and the NHS Executive; they merely jumped onto the band-wagon when it was already moving, coshed the driver and claimed it as theirs.

3.7.4 Achieving quality improvement

Clinical quality
Since it must be health outcomes that primarily interest us as clinical managers, the first concern must be with ensuring high quality of clinical care. Although this is primarily the personal responsibility of clinicians and other professionals, it can be facilitated by management processes:

(1) Ensuring that professionals are properly supported within the organisation and have the facilities with which to do their jobs.
(2) Ensuring that appropriate people are appointed.
(3) Ensuring that supervision is adequate and delegation appropriate.
(4) Ensuring that continuing medical education occurs and that the correct amounts of study and professional leave are taken.
(5) Ensuring that audit is taking place regularly and effectively.
(6) Ensuring that agreed protocols are adhered to.

(7) Ensuring that the job plans are correct for the organisation's needs and that they are adhered to.

There is also the more proactive and general obligation to help the organisation work clinically in the most effective way. The NHS Executive's paper on this describes three components:[15]

(1) *Inform*: i.e. take account of evidence of best practice from whatever source.
(2) *Change* practice to take into account using the evidence.
(3) *Monitor* the results.

One might reasonably add that one must also *reward* the achievement of quality. The award of Charter Marks and various prizes and King's Fund recognitions are all welcome steps in this direction, but more important is giving local publicity and praise for quality improvements when they are achieved.

Risk management
In addition to normal clinical issues there are risk management issues that have a significant impact on clinical outcome, particularly:

(1) The proper supervision of junior staff.
(2) Ensuring continuity of clinical care with proper reporting mechanisms between staff.
(3) Working to ensure that where necessary competent locums are appointed and proper induction procedures are in place for them.

Process improvement
Some quality improvements are dependent on changes in process that need to be both radical and extensive, i.e. stretching along much of the path that the patient takes through the health system. This is only one of many options for quality improvement, but it depends on the contiguous implementation of changes by different teams, thus the medical manager has a central coordinating role to play in commissioning and achieving the improvement.[16] Until recently it was assumed that the patient had no role to play in this, but it is welcome that the new Patient's Charter proposals identify that the patients themselves have obligations and responsibilities to do with communication, attendance, and their attitude to staff.

On becoming involved in radical quality improvement measures, the clinical manager is sure to brush with professional process improvement people. He will need to be aware that, as in EBM and audit, there is a degree of zealatory in them that he may find irritating. If he reads the papers or goes to the meetings he will need only to strip out what is useful without feeling the need to swallow the whole package. Process improvement has become something of an industry, taking its origins from various management fads of the 1970s, 1980s, and 1990s: TQM (total quality management), continuous quality improvement (CQI), business process re-engineering, service quality improvement programmes (SQIP) etc. You'll be told that they are all very different, but in reality they are all much the same. In the Health Service they differ from industry and commerce where they have notoriously been mixed in with "business re-engineering" simply as a vehicle for reducing the size of the workforce. This facet of re-engineering has led to its rebuttal as a business process, but doesn't mean that there are no lessons to learn from it for the NHS.

The least threatening of the publications relating to techniques for use in quality improvement processes is a bulky but practical folder produced by the Department of Health with the imaginative title *Leading Improvement in Health Care—a resource guide for process improvement.*[17]

In essence, the messages about process improvement can be summarised as:

(1) The process of healthcare is currently characterised by good people working in a bad system, not vice versa. More than that the system may be so inept that it requires the heroic efforts of outstanding people in order simply to function.

(2) A system will deliver no more than it is designed to and if a system is flawed it will go wrong regularly.

(3) If you put pressure on a bad system to work better you simply demoralise the people in it and may produce even more problems.

(4) Incremental change and "sticking plaster solutions" are not the way to improve the system; it needs redesign.

(5) A large improvement in quality can be achieved through radical changes in process.

(6) At the working level the NHS exists as parallel functional units, e.g. facilities, medical directorates, surgical directorates,

pathology services, etc. and, at one stage removed, community, GP and ambulance services. All see their own problems and try to fix them themselves. The patient's experience of the system is, however, not vertical but horizontal. Imagine Auntie Flo having a stroke at home and think through the units of the system that sequentially deal with her; GP— hospital switchboard—ambulance—accident and emergency department—medical directorate—stroke unit—social ser- vices—GP; and others in parallel such as speech therapy, physiotherapy, pharmacy, radiology and pathology. There will probably have been no formal communication between these separate units to improve the processes for the Auntie Flos of the world; each separate unit has its own entrenched protocols, usually designed with little reference to those of others.

(7) To rearrange the process to make it work properly needs an analysis of it that is comprehensive and made from the outside; judging the system especially from the patient's point of view. W.E. Deming, the father of quality improvement, talked of the need for "profound knowledge" of the system based on:

(a) knowledge of the system and how the parts interrelate;
(b) knowledge of variation—understanding and measuring the causes of departure from normal so that an action can be taken;
(c) knowledge of psychology to understand why people do what they do;
(d) knowledge of the theory of knowledge—understanding learning processes.

This sounds rather inhibiting as if it excluded the average manager from getting started on the exercise. The average clinical manager, however, needs to understand that she already carries with her an enormous supply of knowledge about clinical medicine and systems; so she is well on the road before she even starts. She also needs to remember that most management theory is common sense jargonised and that she is as likely to be just as able to take the appropriate steps as is a highly paid professional "re-engineer". The analysis of variation merely implies a commitment to identifying the facts of variation; how often does the system not work properly and in what way? The knowledge of psychology is again a basic matter of understanding how to motivate people to embrace change. The last part concerning the theory of knowledge is a rather pretentious way of explaining the concept of continuous change as being a continuing learning process, in which failure is allowed to occur and both success and failure are analysed and built on for the next cycle of change. This is not as comfortable as falling back to the status quo when things go wrong, but is essential to the process of quality improvement. In re-engineering the danger is that you will fix on the process rather than the product, therefore in analysing the system and its failings the users, i.e. staff of all grades and the patients, need to be consulted. The re-engineering exercise in Leicester showed how valuable formally convened panels of these groups can be. The NHS Executive with the King's Fund has undertaken a study of focus groups and confirmed that they do not simply ask for expensive change but tend to fix on cultural and communication issues. Setting up focus groups may however be difficult, and it is not easy to engage ethnic minorities in them.[18]

(8) Having re-engineered the system it is essential regularly to re-visit it and determine whether changes have had the expected results. This is the same cycle as used in audit and the same cycle as described above about learning. The diagram of the cycle is self-evident, but in management books it is grandiosely entitled "The Shewhart PDCA Cycle" (Figure 3.2).

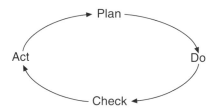

Figure 3.2   The Shewhart PDCA cycle.

3.7.5 The realities of process improvement

Continuous process improvement is different from effective audit. In audit the actions looked at are usually small and closely defined and acting on the results will normally only tinker with the basic process. It is the extensive, radical nature of process re-engineering which makes it difficult for the average institution. Commercial organisations can and *must* afford the huge time, cost and effort needed to re-engineer a process. Hiroshi Harade, President of the Japanese company Ricoh, quoted the cost of correcting a fault in a photocopier at the design stage as $368. To do so before shipment costs $17 000 but after the photocopier was in the hands of the customers it cost $590 000. One might think that savings in the Health Service are either not there or of a totally different scale. That is true for individual trusts but may be not for the whole organisation, and the end point is "improved customer satisfaction" rather than a "cheaper product". Process re-engineering is time consuming and if outside consultants are brought in to help it is also very expensive (the exercises at King's College Hospital and Leicester Royal Infirmary cost millions of pounds). If in-house managers are used then the other work of the organisation suffers. So contrary to the professional re-engineer's vigorous support of radical change as the means of improving quality, there is much to be said for undertaking re-engineering in bite-sized pieces—the development of one-stop clinics is a good example. You may find common factors that obstruct the development of a smooth-running service such as archaic booking systems, difficult access to radiology, slow pathology reporting, and absent notes. A focus group of patients will identify problems that you did not know you had. These specifics will need to be addressed in the first re-engineering project, but then make subsequent projects very much easier. For example the depressing (for the patients) problem of long waits and queues in outpatients can sometimes be tackled by the application of computerised "Decision Support Systems" which can show how best to reconfigure the booking system to avoid delays. The principles and the software are applicable in many different queuing situations.[19] The problem is that in doing such an analysis, and indeed in almost all such projects, money is required at start-up. The examples listed above mostly need expenditure to put them right. The enthusiasts for re-engineering say that the improvement process results in a new system which costs less to run and is more productive, although it is difficult to find examples to confirm this. The absence of start-up money has sadly led to many worthwhile projects being suffocated at birth, and is another symptom of the short-termism and compartmentalisation of NHS financing. In fairness to the ever wary director of finance, one must add that

74

the finances often turn out not just to be "start-up" money, and for true quality improvement a number of costs will continue. For example in my own experience of re-engineering a "one-stop clinic", it was found necessary to up-grade the salaries of the clerks to attract people of sufficient quality and to employ clinical assistants to bring down the waiting times to a manageable level. Extra equipment had to be found to enable a cytologist to work within the clinic. Most of the time and effort, however, was simply establishing a written protocol and persuading colleagues in other departments to change their working practices.

The unwillingness explicitly to commit finance to projects that have quality gain rather than an identifiable health gain have tempted management to use a back-door route to quality improvement, a shabby manoeuvre all too common in the Health Service. The technique is simply to demand improved quality standards as part of a commissioning process or as part of the establishment of a league table or recognition process, then to police them aggressively but not to provide any help to assist in their achievement. The purchaser/provider split and the need for service specifications has been the perfect vehicle for this kind of exercise, and as the process engineers would have predicted it often merely leads to the process corrupting itself artificially to produce the required data implying that the quality has occurred when in fact it has not.

3.7.6 Quality assessment

The assessment of quality is in essence what audit is all about, and the definition of audit given in "Working for Patients" is "the systematic, critical analysis of the *quality* of medical care, including the procedures used for diagnosis and treatment, the use of resources and the resulting outcome and *quality* of life for the patient".[20] Audit will be discussed elsewhere in this book. What concerns us here is what quality measures the medical manager can and should audit and what are the motives for requiring him to do that. Maxwell's parameters of quality in healthcare mark out the areas which need to be assessed and improved: *Effectiveness, Efficiency, Appropriateness, Acceptability, Access,* and *Equity.*[21]

As clinicians we are concerned with the quality experienced by individual patients and are clear that the quality is in two parts:

(1) *The process* should be as pleasing as possible to the patient; this is about access, communication, courtesy, privacy, environment, etc.

and

(2) *The outcome* which should be as good as possible, i.e. there should be appropriate care for maximum health gain with minimum disbenefit.

As managers we also wish to ensure that we are running a high-quality organisation in the business sense, optimally productive and cost effective. The assessment of business quality should not be confused with the assessment of clinical quality, and the achievement of the latter may, of course, be at the expense of the former. In commercial organisations, of course, high-quality service in the sense of process is crucial to the well being of a competitive organisation in the open market. In a normal market the pressures of consumerism are constructive. One is not supposed to mention it, but in the NHS consumerist pressures rarely focus on the real issues of health outcome instead they may be a distraction, focusing predominantly on process and comfort issues. Thus in using their time and energy to assess quality outcomes, medical managers need to have a clear list of priorities:

(1) health outcome
(2) process quality
(3) cost effectiveness.

You could argue that because poor cost effectiveness can take away money needed for achieving health gain, it should take precedence over quality of process. Either way the current problem is the obsession with measuring (2) and (3) to the exclusion of (1), and the problem is also to do with motive which is as much to do with a desire for control as a desire to improve. The medical manager may also find irritating the insistence on continuous monitoring rather than on sampling, even though the continuous monitoring of data is expensive of resources and frustrating for staff. Unfortunately the monitoring of health outcome is the most difficult.

Monitoring health outcomes
This does not mean that only end points need to be measured. If quality control exercises improve the accuracy of cervical cytology

or mammography or reduce infection or the need for re-admission, then it is reasonable to assume that there is an impact on the all important health gain end point.

Everyone wants information on clinical outcomes. These measures have an intuitive appeal: high-quality care should be reflected by good outcomes therefore, poorer outcomes should indicate deficiencies in care, including missed opportunities or wasted resources. The hope is that data on outcomes will provide a barometer for health care, indicating the effectiveness and efficiency of service delivery.[22]

However the measurement of clinical outcome is a very inexact science. Unfortunately some measures can be deceptively informative. Even the easiest outcome to measure, death, the number of patients having treatment who die, is only meaningful when compared to an exactly comparable population. The effects of case-mix routinely frustrate interpretation, except in rare instances of sophisticated systems such as APACHE II for scoring ITU patients. Studies on treatments that are, or could be, multimodal show that even quite wide ranges of quality in the application of these treatments have minimal effects on measurable outcome in the short term.[23] Purchasers' measures of effectiveness and government league tables which ignore case-mix and statistics are worse than useless, giving spurious honour to those whom population bias, case selection and statistical serendipity have thrust to the top of the list. For the government to use meaningless "league tables" in a widely publicised "naming and shaming" exercise is not simply an unfortunate reflection on their intellectual credulity but a tragedy when all it does is seed widespread anxiety into the very populations they are claiming to act for.

The publication of league tables does however change behaviour, although it may not do so in the way intended. In some states of the USA death rates after cardiac surgery are published and the effects of this have been studied. Some surgeons with poor outcomes and low operating volumes stopped operating but few other changes in practice or outcome were noted. However it became more difficult to get poor risk patients operated upon and the database changed as more attention was paid to recording co-morbidity, etc.[24] It is a statistical minefield fit only for trained public health clinicians, it is not what it is at present, a playground for politicians. Comparative studies of outcome are crucial and facilitating the data collection, assessing the results and acting upon them will be a major role for clinical managers in the future. Public health doctors are well aware of the difficulties in the process of establishing clinical effectiveness indicators. The first stab at this activity has produced an odd looking list of 14 indicators, which includes the obvious candidates like MMR immunisation rates and breast and cervical screening coverage. The list also includes quirky things like Statin prescribing in general practice for which there is no agreed standard, cochlear implant rates where the numbers are so small as to be statistically meaningless, and hip and knee replacements where previous good performance will produce spuriously "poor" performance now. But never mind, as long as we all keep a sense of clinical and statistical reality about us the process will be valuable quite apart from providing a lifetime of gainful employment for public health physicians.

For the moment the measurement of process is normally our best mechanism for predicting rather than measuring outcome and thus quality of care, but it does require that we measure quality by degree of adherence to very clearly defined and agreed standards. Unfortunately these are only available in a limited number of clinical instances. For example, the percentage of premenopausal women with node-positive breast cancer receiving chemotherapy or the percentage of patients with myocardial infarction receiving thrombolysis within 6 hours. Medical managers need to make clear judgments about the validity of the criteria which are going to be used as "gold standards" of quality. This in turn leads back not only to the validity of EBM as a process but also to an awareness that bureaucratisation of the process can lead to the original measure being misrepresented or inappropriate. For example, concerning the management of breast cancer, when breast conserving surgery is used a second re-excision of the area surrounding the tumour may be needed to achieve "clear margins". Recently purchasers' questionnaires have asked for the percentage of re-operative specimens containing residual tumour. These answers are uninterpretable without a knowledge of other variables about the patient which are not collected. Furthermore, the question itself is predicated on the assumption that clear margins are essential, a view not supported by all the data. In this example a simple bureaucratic mechanism has attempted to distil a very complex clinical process and in doing so has lost its power. A powerful and valid test is one in which many questions are proposed, answers received in a pilot study are correlated with the desired end point, in this case quality, and then only those questions which correlated closely are asked in future. This is a familiar technique to psychologists but an alien concept it seems to many managers. In the case of poor quality breast surgery we know the features of those surgeons and centres who have been shown to have poor outcomes.[25,26] The two main correlates are, firstly, seeing only a few patients and, second, having no regular contact with medical oncologists. The enthusiasts for collecting every tiny bit of data about breast surgical services need to prove that they can do better than simply acting on those two pieces of relevant data which they already have. Collecting data is of course infinitely easier than acting on data.

There are many dangers inherent in these extensive data collection processes. The first and rarely tested criticism is that they are simply not a cost-effective addition to our means of improving peoples' health. Second, when the data collection is inflicted on people who do not themselves need it and do not respect the motives of those who demand it, the data are unlikely to be valid. Worse than that a new form of defensive medicine develops. The rejection of poor risk patients is a serious but probably overemphasised example of this. A more classic example is the "Hello Nurse" in the accident and emergency department employed solely to greet and quickly assess the patients as they come through the door in order that all patients can be said, for the purposes of quality standards, to have been assessed within 5 minutes. In reality the majority will then wait just as long as they ever did to be properly assessed or treated.

The tragedy of the obsession with monitoring is that it is a declaration of failure. We should be expending our efforts on picking, training, supporting and rewarding people so that we do not have to monitor their performance all the time. This is not Utopian, it is simply a different philosophy about managing of people and processes.

It has been claimed that there is a pervading culture that "Quality is asserted not measured".[27] We do need "quality control" but it must involve:

- Parameters agreed by all parties as meaningful. One should be sure to avoid "The MacNamara Fallacy", so we must seek to measure what is important not make important what we can measure.

- Parameters agreed by all parties as useful.
- Measurable parameters.
- Parameters assessable by sampling rather than continuous measurement.
- An acceptance that professionals within the service will act professionally.
- A guarantee that the data is not used out of context.

3.7.7 Clinical governance

The 1997 White Paper "The New NHS, Modern and Dependable" identified an area for attention which it called "clinical governance", which is a term whose interpretation is of the government's own making for the words themselves tell us nothing much. Governance can mean either "the act of governing" or "the state of being governed",[28] but the new phrase is all about maintaining standards and appears to mean a process driven from above whereby all the threads that contribute to quality of care are drawn together in the organisation facilitated, monitored and policed. Nationally there will be a Commission for Health Improvement (CHIMP) and a National Institute for Clinical Effectiveness (NICE!).[29] At trust and hospital level someone on the board, probably the medical director, will need to oversee a systematic process which will:

- Ensure the continuous improvement in the quality of professional and clinical services provided by the organisation.
- Encourage and guide the dissemination of good practice.
- Evaluate, support and monitor clinical practice.
- Facilitate the rapid detection and open investigation of adverse incidents and ensure that lessons are learnt from them.

The principle is worthy, the need I suppose self-evident, though it is yet another instance of an official belief that professionals are incapable of fulfilling these tasks themselves and must be chivvied into them. Nobody really knows whether the effort that will be required will be justified. In the management parlance will there be any "added value" or will it be just a further extension of the existing bureaucracy?

The spectrum of activities that will need to be tied together is daunting. It will include quality initiatives, risk management, audit, EBM, educational strategies, new technology, introduction of new drugs, Continuing Professional Development (CPD), Continuing

Medical Education (CME), the Patient's Charter, New Deal compliance, accreditation, complaints, poor performance enquiries, and so on. More things will need to be photocopied, more committees will need to redigest regurgitated products of other digestions, more convoluted guidance documents will be issued and, unless the process is carried out extremely sensitively, those in the front line will again feel undermined and untrusted and the process will be seen simply as a political exercise and another facet of the central obsession with control in the NHS.

If the process is managed delicately it may indeed help professionals to "do the right thing" and "do it the right way", and if it is to be handled well, the medical director and clinical directors will need to be deeply involved. It is certainly not going to be possible to escape the process, as trusts will carry a statutory duty of quality assurance following changes in the law planned for 1999.

What will the medical manager need to do?

When the grim-faced person from CHIMP comes to visit the Medical Director of Slapdash and Poorly Healthtrust, she will probably be wanting to know something which the board of any trust should already know:

(1) Are you ensuring that your organisation is using best practice?
(2) Are you educating your staff to achieve that?
(3) Are you monitoring your outcomes to ensure that they are satisfactory?
(4) Do you have the right culture and procedures to ensure that you respond promptly to anxieties about poor performance?
(5) Are complaints dealt with correctly and the lessons from them spread through the organisation to encourage appropriate changes in practice?
(6) Do you have a formal structure in place for assessing and minimising clinical risk and is there a critical incident reporting system in place?
(7) Do you have a means of exploring opportunities for quality improvement in different service areas?

She will probably ask: "Will you show me the documentation that confirms all this and let me have a copy of the annual report in which it is summarised?" You might be tempted to retort that, particularly for the educational, monitoring and collation exercises, there are large unmet costs of implementation and there are significant administrative costs. You will probably be tempted to ask her from where you are expected to find that funding. She will no doubt smile very sweetly and reply that the exercise is intended to be "cost neutral".

In response to all this you may be very tempted to give the issue very low priority, but you should not. The unhappy saga of the bad results from paediatric cardiac surgical care at Bristol which unfurled themselves across the newspapers between the autumn of 1997 and the summer of 1998 underline the responsibilities that clinical managers have to act in the face of data showing poor quality. Doctors who are managers, and that included in the Bristol case the chief executive who was a doctor, were judged to be reprehensible because the data were said clearly to indicate poor performance, and yet the management side failed to act. We will never know whether the outcome would have been different if the current initiatives on clinical governance had occurred 5 years ago. If the culture of an organisation is wrong it needs more than directives from the NHS Executive to put it right.

If clinical managers see themselves as the agents of good quality and sound practice, rather than policemen guarding the trust's financial bottom line, then they have nothing to fear from clinical governance.

At the end of all this one wonders if all the paperwork and the exhortations and inspection committees are not actually missing the point that the real guarantors of quality are motivated, committed, supported professionals within the service, and that much of what has happened over the last 10 years has damaged rather than enhanced the motivation and commitment of those professionals. But maybe I'm wrong about that, it's not easy to measure.

3.8 Communicating

One of the maxims of management that is almost true is that you cannot communicate too much or too often. The single most important function of the clinician in management is as a communicator. He is the two-way channel between the management and the clinical staff and his grounding in patient care should also help to optimise the communication the organisation has with its patients. The realities of NHS medicine will also involve him in communicating with the media.

3.8.1 Communications with colleagues

Your achievements as a practical manager and leader and your ability to get things done will depend on your communications skills; firstly as a listener and, secondly, as a transmitter. The simplest way to do all this is to retreat to your office, wait for the letters and telephone calls as your input and spend your time dictating letters, e-mails and position papers as your output. There is a beguiling roundness about a completed paper or letter, a reassuring finality about pressing the button to send off the e-mail, but there is a truly Faustian risk that the process can become the end in itself, enabling you to avoid the hard grind of personal contact. Also it too easily fits the traditional pattern of Health Service management where a lot of messages are sent down the line but they pass very few coming up. Within the confines of a hospital communication is better served by face-to-face contact; don't write—visit; don't send a circular—discuss at a team meeting; don't just look at the balance sheet and the productivity graphs—go walkabout. For managers face-to-face contact involves difficult balancing acts between listening and influencing and between promising and refusing. The psychologists like to refer to these contacts as "transactions" and where they are in relation to conflict they are discussed in Sections 4.3 and 4.6. In the more normal day-to-day transaction it is important to remember that the psychologists' claim that 38% of non-technical, face-to-face messages are carried by the voice/tone inflection and 55% by outward behaviour such as body language, dress and size. This leaves only a paltry 7% to be carried by the words. This theory leaves you with a problem if you are 5 feet 2 inches tall with a stutter, though one excellent manager of my acquaintance, seriously handicapped and barely 4 feet tall, manages everybody from the grumpiest clinician to the most intransigent porter simply by force of character. If there's a problem perhaps your communication skills would be improved by an assertiveness or communication course, however I doubt it as communication skills seem to be inherent rather than learnt.

"Walkabouts", visits to a specific area announced or unannounced, pose an interesting range of problems. They are time consuming and they commit you to a barrage of invalidated facts and opinions. You will probably have noticed how books for armchair travellers fix not on general descriptions of places but on quirky little observations and incidents which are felt to reveal the true character of the place. So too with walkabouts where the truth may sometimes seem to be encapsulated in a chance remark from a cleaner, but beware of your own susceptibility to such persuasive vignettes and check them later against hard facts.

Team meetings with consultants have a tendency to be disappointing. Consultants are by nature not malleable team players, and even if they come to meetings they have difficulty in responding as equals when nurses and junior managers are present, though one hopes that this is becoming a thing of the past.

3.8.2 Communication throughout the organisation

This is more difficult. Indeed, the size and mix of the audience makes it impossible to communicate equally effectively with everybody. Some managers, on the assumption that the more communicating you do the better, flood the place with paperwork, none personalised and much of it too general to be of interest to the average reader. Doctors in particular are inundated with unsolicited paper both at home and at work, so if communications are not to end up in the bin they need to be targeted carefully. Observations suggest that some or all of the following formats are worth considering:

(1) Trust-wide regular information sheets included with the medical advisory committee minutes or in payslip packets.

(2) Regular concise information for all staff, in newspaper format if the organisation is large enough. Modern computerised desktop publishing packages make this cheap and easy. A separate paper for doctors is worthwhile; it might include impending appointments, details of new appointees, time-tables of educational events, changes in service availability (e.g. closure of laboratories over holidays), and "plain-speak" summaries of topics of current interest. The British Association of Medical Managers issues such "plain-speak" summaries to its members.

(3) Wallposters for urgent and very important issues. These can summarise the message in a couple of hundred words of large type on a sheet of A3 paper in such a way that almost everyone in the organisation can be aware of the message within the day. The wording is, of course, critical as there is no supporting literature. The message must be explicit.

(4) Team briefing papers. I know of one hospital which has generic summaries produced by the executive at its meetings. These are printed down one side of the page. Each directorate then adds its own comments about relevance or action plans in the broad margin before circulating photocopies to the team.

(5) A central reference point for the bulky and the boring kilos of reports and directives that reach the hospital each month from the NHS Executive, regions, royal colleges and educational bodies etc. It helps if these are properly documented and cross-referenced and summaries available.

(6) One hope is that in the future much more use of hospital computer systems will be made particularly those linked to the NHS network, so as to mimic the Internet. My trust already has access on its ward terminals to the medical database Medline, to hospital protocols, clinical advice, telephone numbers and the house officers' handbook, in addition to e-mail and access to the normal information about beds, lab. results, etc. Soon then, staff will be able to "surf" the hospital net to obtain all the information they need. Unfortunately that means that they will need to know what it is they need to know!

To avoid security problems hospital computers are not normally connected to the Internet but the new NHS net may provide adequate "firewalls" to allow it, thus opening up to staff not only the oceans of information to which patients have access but also allowing them their own Web sites. If you are on the Internet already try:

- http://www.york.ac.uk/inst/crd/welcome.htm for the NHS Centre for Reviews and Dissemination.
- http://www.open.gov.uk/doh/dhhome.htm for the DHSS.
- http://www.nahat.net for The National Association of Health Authorities and Trusts (NAHAT).
- http:www.omni.ac.uk and http://www.medmatrix.org for research into clinical topics.

It is difficult to know whether to recommend the copious productions of national bodies as a model of communications. No doubt they are professionally planned and indeed their advisory documents on audit, evidence-based medicine, re-engineering, etc. are models of clear language, explicit advice and elegant presentation. These are a marked contrast to the densely typed productions on non-glossy paper which outline new legislation. The "orange book" defining the Calman training proposals is one such example,[30] the very user unfriendliness of which must have set back the process substantially. The Executive Letters, now called NHS Circulars, that direct our lives, while brief, have all the presentational charm of an EEC directive on the texture of meatballs. The last lesson to learn from centrally produced documents can be seen in newsletters. There is a unique naffness about their exhortatory style, presenting only accounts of success or imagined success larded with head and shoulders photographs of people we have never met and produced on expensive, glossy paper that our unfunded, hand-illustrated, photocopied handouts to patients can never hope to match.

3.8.3 The volume of paperwork

In 1995 the Department of Health is estimated to have sent out:[31]

- over a million pages to trusts and health authorities
- over 300 management letters
- about 400 other publications to health authorities
- around 200 other publications to trusts.

In 1995, Stephen Dorrell the then Secretary of State, set up an investigation into the means by which this volume might be reduced. The report of that investigation[32] concluded that the problem was more widespread than the figures above suggest. The British Association of Medical Managers (BAMM) ran a parallel survey[33] and concluded that the main culprits were:

- In trusts: the business planning process.
- Commissioning: too many and duplicated requests for data.
- Centrally (the NHS Executive is the major culprit in all this): too many directives, consultation documents and requests for data without prioritisation or targeting.
- The fact that the whole system is paper based.

The solutions proposed were clearly vehicles for clinical managers to express many of their frustrations with NHS bureaucracy. Among other things they proposed:

- Improved electronic communications.
- Targeted mailing.
- Authors made to draft all communications in longhand.
- Nothing to be longer than one page of A4 paper.
- Doing away with inappropriate, repetitive and spurious monitoring and data collection exercises.
- Charges for the provision of data.
- Halving the number of people employed by purchasers.
- Reducing the amount of legislation applied to the NHS.
- Reducing central control and increasing the autonomy of trusts.
- Etc., etc.

The summary makes very cheery reading, confirming a communality of complaint among clinical directors which does not normally find a platform.

The Department of Health did respond to the "Seeing the Wood, Sparing the Trees" initiative, and in 1998 changed from the habit of multiple types of management letter to a single series called "Health Service Circulars". This will be available electronically at http://www.open.gov.uk/doh/coinh.htm. As yet, though, there is not much evidence of a reduction in the quantity of paperwork issued nor can one realistically expect this for as long as the NHS remains centrally managed by design, anxious by inclination and prescriptive by habit. The "Seeing The Wood, Sparing the Trees" paper commented that "developing a more mature relationship, based on openness and trust would be the single most important move towards minimizing bureaucracy".

3.8.4 Communicating with the public

The NHS communicates ineptly with the public. Take for example the public meeting. NHS trusts are required to have public meetings to present themselves and their results and these meetings can be the ultimate example of a hollow communication exercise. It has been calculated that about 1 in 10 000 to 1 in 100 000 of the users of services attend the meetings, usually the embittered opponents of change, local politicians, ideological zealots, and a little old lady with a string bag who is the only person who comes to listen rather than speak. The fare is often a carefully crafted best-view of the organisation's achievements and the whole event can quickly descend into farce once the questions begin. It is symbolic of the impotence of the public to challenge accountability within the Health Service. Public meetings to debate changes proposed in NHS facilities are organised by the local commissioning health authority, and the difficulty here is that there are rarely two or more options, the choice between which will genuinely depend on public preference. The views of those attending the meetings and those presenting at them are equally well known and the value of the exercise very limited other than to remind the players how uncomfortable change can be. The present government's intention to open trust board meetings to the public is hardly likely *ipso facto* to change the relationships into something more constructive. Managers who manage to set up a calm, apolitical, constructive two-way communication channel with their patients will have done a great service.

3.8.5 Communicating through the media

There are great dangers in trying to use the media as a vehicle for manipulating rather than communicating, because it is so unpredictable and unreliable. It is, however, an unfortunate reality that the upward channels to the NHS Executive and the government are so tenuous that often only pressure from the media has any impact. Health stories are part of their stock-in-trade, readily carried without much attempt at checking the facts or putting them in context, partly one suspects because of the corrupting effect of deadlines and the desire for a scoop. Bricks can indeed be made without straw if they need only last a day or two. The transparently inaccurate or overstated items display an eerie lack of basic knowledge about medicine; for example on 6 June 1997 both *The Independent* and *The Daily Mail* announced that "Australian scientists have developed the first nano-machine which will enable doctors to provide an instant diagnosis of virtually all known diseases". More subtle and more damaging is the cavalier attitude to statistics, such that for instance in 1997 the public were told that the risk of breast cancer for those on hormone replacement therapy is "2.3 times higher or more than double that of non users". In fact the *Lancet* article on which that headline was based identifies the relative risk as a paltry 1.023.[34,35] If efforts are not made to counterbalance the inherent naivety and imbalance of media stories, real damage to patients can be done. For example data from the Office of

National Statistics showed an unexpected 14 000 rise in legal abortions in 1996 in England and Wales, which was attributed to women precipitately stopping oral contraception after scare stories about the safety of oral contraceptives in 1995. This was however an improvement on the 50 000 extra unplanned pregnancies that occurred after a similar scare story in 1969. These problems are not just the fault of the media. C.P. Snow's *Two Cultures and the Scientific Revolution* was published in 1959 and the gulf which it identified between science (which includes medical science) and the rest of the world has widened since then. Susan Okie, a medical journalist on the *Washington Post*, has written about the declining scientific literacy of journalists and the deteriorating general literacy of doctors and scientists and how this widens the communication gulf.[36] Doctors have got to spend much more time learning how to explain to the media as well as to the patients what they're up to. For all that the medical manager needs to be practiced or cautious in her dealings with the media. This is particularly so when she becomes embroiled with the press over an unexpected crisis. A major accident in your catchment area is simply time consuming, but an apparently straightforward clinical decision can turn into public relations nightmare as the "child B" case exemplified. Child B was a child under the care of the Cambridgeshire and Huntingdon Health Authority; relapsing yet again from her leukaemia she was judged not to be an appropriate candidate for a second marrow transplant. The Extra Contractual Referral was refused but the father used the willing press as the vehicle for his protest at this. The health authority and the clinicians involved were thus immediately cast as the villains, a situation difficult to retrieve even with the most practised public relations; something which most trusts simply do not have. One option is for such trusts to use external PR agencies. One agency covers 30 trusts and health authorities, giving 24-hour cover. NHS trusts have been criticised for employing public relations people, and where they function simply as salesmen for trusts in a commercial market context one can understand that criticism. They do, however, spend more time explaining the trusts' activities to local people and the press, and by softening the hard edge that exists between hospitals and the world outside must surely be worthwhile.

A useful list of "fright factors" and "media triggers" appears in Table 3.1.

Table 3.1 "Fright factors" and "media triggers": things that are particularly likely to lead to media coverage of a medical story

Fright factors	Media triggers
Risks are generally more worrying (and less acceptable) if perceived: 1. To be involuntary (such as exposure to a pollutant) rather than voluntary (e.g. dangerous sports or smoking) 2. As inequitably distributed (some benefit while others suffer the consequences) 3. As inescapable by taking personal precautions 4. To arise from an unfamiliar or novel source 5. To result from man-made, rather than natural sources 6. To cause hidden and irreversible damage (e.g. through onset of illness many years after exposure) 7. To pose some particular danger to small children or pregnant women or more generally to future generations 8. To threaten a form of death (or illness/injury) arousing particular dread 9. To damage identifiable rather than anonymous victims 10. To be poorly understood by science 11. As subject to contradictory statements from responsible sources (or, even worse, from the same source)	A possible risk to public health is more likely to become a major story if the following are prominent or can readily be made to become so: 1. Questions of blame 2. Alleged secrets and attempted "cover-ups" 3. "Human interest" through identifiable heroes, villains, dupes etc. (as well as victims) 4. Links with existing high-profile issues (or personalities) 5. Conflict (including conflict between experts, and between experts and public) 6. Signal value: the story as a portent of further or more general ills e.g.: the inadequacy of regulatory controls. ("What next?") 7. Many people exposed to the risk even if at low levels ("It could be you!") 8. Strong visual impact 9. Sex and/or crime 10. Reference back to other reports: the fact that something is a "story" is often itself a story, creating a snowball effect as media compete for coverage

(Reproduced from: Rodwell L. A matter of perspective. *NHS Magazine* 1998;**12**:11)

3.8.6 Communicating information to patients

We are not good at communicating information to patients. The brevity of consultations, the habits of paternalistic medicine combine with a norm that non-medical staff do not give out medical facts and leave most patients in an information desert. Under pressure from patients things are improving and the burgeoning alternative sources of information on the Internet, in leaflets, books and magazines challenges us to orchestrate the production of relevant, comprehensible and accurate material for patients. Much of what is currently given out is of very poor quality and could be improved by adherence to checklists that can be used to enhance the quality.[37] In relation to the Internet there is a particular urgency about this, as even the briefest of acquaintance with the 10 000 health-related websites will show much of it to be inaccurate, commercial, personalised, irrelevant, out of date, or just plain weird. Entertaining but not what is needed. One study of the accuracy of the Internet looked at advice on managing fever in children at home. Forty-one pages were found but only four adhered to published guidelines.[38]

Open telephone enquiry lines are seen as a good way of offering appropriate information, and the government is currently establishing telephone helplines manned by ambulance personnel or nurses. The concept is good but large numbers of appropriately trained staff will need to be recruited. Ready access to "Hello, this is the Health Hotline, my name is Deirdre, how can I help you? . . ." will be a triumph in itself, but managers will need to be clear about the function of such lines. In the USA they are used for "demand management" as a way of helping people to use health care resources wisely. We will need to measure whether that could be effective here and learn who should supervise and staff them.

The budgets needed for communications with patients have often been missing in the past, but in the future medical managers will need to make sure that not only is information made available before, during and after peoples' contact with hospitals, but that the information is consistent with what actually happens. The impending arrival of very crude and potentially misleading league tables is likely to add impetus to hospitals' need to communicate the real facts to its patients.

References

1 Simpson T, Scott T. *Leading Clinical Services*. The British Association of Medical Managers, 1997.
2 Council of International Hospitals. *The Role of the Clinical Director*, 1997, October.
3 The Association of Trust Medical Directors. *The Role and Responsibility of the Medical Director*. British Association of Medical Managers, 1996.
4 Rivett G. *From Cradle to Grave*. London: King's Fund 1998.
5 Bradshaw A. Charting some challenges in the art and science of nursing. *Lancet* 1998;**351**:438–40.
6 Quail M. Nurse executive's pay: a survey for the Royal College of Nursing. *Health Serv J* 1997; 9 January:9. (See also Motivation and

satisfaction among nurse executive directors in NHS Trusts. Royal College of Nursing.)

7 Kakabadse A. *Wealth Creators*. London: Kogan Page, 1992.

8 Caplan RP. Stress, anxiety and depression in hospital consultants, general practitioners and senior health service managers. *Br Med J* 1994;**309**:1261–3.

9 Institute of Work Psychology, University of Sheffield. Cited in *The Observer* 15 March 1998.

10 Kent G, Johnson AG. Conflicting demands in surgical practice. *Ann R Coll Surg Engl* 1995;**77** (Suppl):235–8.

11 Cited in "Style section", *The Sunday Times* 1997;23 March:39.

12 Howard P. *Weasel Words*. London: Hamish Hamilton, 1978.

13 Hurst DK. Business planning. In: Hurst DK, Clements RV, eds. *Clinical Director's Handbook*. London: Churchill Livingstone, 1995, p. 46.

14 Caulkin S. Interview with Stainton J. *The Observer* 1997; 9 October (and of course many others!).

15 NHS Excutive. *Promoting Clinical Effectiveness*. London: Department of Health, 1996.

16 Berwick DM, Enthoven A, Bunker JP. Quality management in the NHS: the doctor's role. *Br Med J* 1992;**304**:304–8.

17 NHS Executive, Department of Health. *Leading Improvement in Health Care—a resource guide for process improvement*. London: HMSO, June 1995.

18 Long-term Medical Conditions Alliance. *Patients Influencing Purchasers*. NHS Confederation, 1997.

19 Worthington D. Queue management. In: Cropper S, Forte P, eds. *Enhancing Health Services Management*. Milton Keynes, Buckinghamshire: Open University Press, 1997, pp. 177–98.

20 Department of Health. *Working for Patients*. Working Paper 6, Command 555. London: HMSO, 1989.

21 Maxwell R. Quality assessment in health. *Br Med J* 1984;**288**:1470–2.

22 Davies HTO, Crombie IK. Assessing the quality of care. *Br Med J* 1995;**311**:766.

23 Mant J, Hicks N. Detecting differences in quality of care; the sensitivity of measures of process and outcome in treating acute myocardial infarction. *Br Med J* 1995;**311**:793–7.

24 McKee M. Indicators of poor clinical performance. *Br Med J* 1997; **315**:142.

25 Salisbury R *et al*. Influence of clinician workload and patterns of treatment on survival from breast cancer. *Lancet* 1995;**354**:1265–70.

26 Gillis CR, Hole DJ. Survival outcome of care by specialist surgeons in breast cancer. *Br Med J* 1996;**312**:145–7.

27 Spiers J. *The Invisible Hospital and the Secret Garden*. Oxford: Radcliffe Medical Press, 1995, p. 50.

28 *Longman's Dictionary of Contemporary English*. London: Longmans, 1978.

29 Department of Health. *A First Class Service: quality in the new NHS*. Health Service Circular HSC(98) 113. London: HMSO, 1998.

30 NHS Executive. *A Guide to Specialist Registrar Training.* London: Department of Health, 1995.
31 NAHAT Briefing Paper. No 99, June 1996.
32 NHS Executive. *Seeing the Wood, Sparing the Trees.* London: Department of Health, 1996.
33 Simpson J. The burden of excessive paperwork in the NHS. *Clinician in Management* 1996;**5**:5–7.
34 Horton R. ICRF from mayhem to meltdown. *Lancet* 1997;**350**:1043–4.
35 Abbasi K. Headlines: more perilous than pills. *Br Med J* 1998;**316**:82.
36 Okie SM. Behind the headlines. *Harvard Med Alumni Bull* 1998;**72**:22–4.
37 Jadad AR, Gagliardi A. Rating health information on the Internet: navigating to knowledge or to Babel? *Lancet* 1998;**279**:611–14.
38 Impicciatore P *et al.* Reliability of health information for the public on the World Wide Web. *Br Med J* 1997;**314**:1875–81.

4 Managing People

Doctors tend to think they are good at managing people because they are doctors but it does not follow. In the course of normal work a doctor's normal interpersonal relationships are fourfold:

(1) With patients.
(2) With his team.
(3) With colleagues.
(4) With friends.

(1) and (2) are highly structured hierarchical relationships in which the doctor is the acknowledged dominant partner. (3) and (4) are primarily peer relationships in which the skills are social and do not much involve inspiring, leading, persuading, negotiating, managing conflict, or delegating, skills central to the management role because managers have to get things done through others.

In spite of the social handicaps of their professional experience, doctors are in my experience no better and no worse than managers at deploying these special skills, which are mostly innate or learned informally. These skills are in fact so difficult to teach that one needs to choose clinical managers who can come to the job with the skills in place.

Specific tasks when managing people

- Getting the best out of people.
- Building a team/making appointments.
- Managing conflict.
- Dealing with contracts and job descriptions.
- Rewarding staff.
- Managing difficult colleagues/disciplinary issues.
- Sick doctors.
- Arranging and monitoring personal and professional development.

4.1 Getting the best out of individuals

Management texts like to start by quoting MacGregor's X and Y theories about the motivation of people at work. Theory X suggests that people are lazy, would rather not work, and will only do so when coerced. Furthermore the average person wishes to be told what to do and if she has personal security will be content. Theory Y suggests that people actually find work stimulating and satisfying and have an inherent capacity to work towards objectives. Furthermore most have an untapped capacity to take the initiative with problems and be responsible for achieving targets. Individuals gain the greatest satisfaction through achieving these targets.

Management texts then suggest that there lurks a Y person in every X person waiting to be brought out by good management. This smacks somewhat of Christian notions of original sin and the possibility of redemption through love but appeals as a modus operandi. Rather more cynically one should perhaps accept that the concepts define not just two possible types of worker but caricature two stereotypes of workers imagined by managers. Most people, of course, have a bit of theory X in them and a bit of theory Y, and need to be managed accordingly in the hope of being moved entirely into the Y configuration.

Although the principles of getting the best out of people are well known and consistent through management teachings, it is sad how many people in the Health Service are made unhappy not by the major and intractable problems of the service but by local irritants and bad person-to-person management. Human relationships are indeed the real tragedies of life. When managing people the touchstones of success may be:

- To include them in the team.
- To understand their informal cultural relationships with you and with their peers (not easy if you're a doc.).
- To set them clear and achievable targets, ideally as a joint exercise.
- To provide constructive feedback and to recognise achievement freely.
- To support them in times of difficulty.
- To reward them appropriately.
- To allow them opportunities to develop new skills.

If all this is done well the employee will, in theory, share the team's purpose, be loyal, motivated, and at the end of the day

95

content. Interestingly financial reward is not seen to be as important in all this as you would expect. If you wish to see these truths in action in your own hospital I suggest you look at the nurses.

Nurses are a very mobile labour force familiar with voting with their feet, so you can learn a lot by finding which areas in the hospital attract nurses and which areas have high turnover and vacancy problems—then gently look for the reasons. A Royal College of Nursing survey in 1997 showed that NHS trusts are suffering a 21% turnover among nursing staff each year and that 65% of nurses report that they worked longer hours then they are contracted, much of it unpaid. But if your organisation troubles to find out from those leaving the exact reasons for their doing so (by using exit interviews or questionnaires), you will find that it is often because of:

- Unachievable workloads due to failure to set or recruit to a realistic establishment.
- Unsympathetic ward sisters or managers.
- Because there are no opportunities for professional development.
- Because they believe they have been graded unfairly.

Almost all these reflect on the management skills brought to bear on them—or lack of management skills.

4.1.1 Supporting staff

You can judge a company by the people it keeps.

(Advertisement for Microsoft Corporation)

If you are a clinical director or medical director you are effectively an employer in the eyes of the team. You have it in your gift to be a good employer or otherwise. This has nothing to do with your training as a manager, it is the human stance that you take and as a doctor a hard, financially driven attitude to your staff is less likely to be forgiven than it might be in a non-clinical manager. You will not be forgiven if in cahoots with the nurse manager you try to make savings by setting unrealistically low staffing levels or insist on inappropriate skill mixes. In managing individuals the particular areas in which your response can be kindly and humane include particularly sickness leave and maternity leave; both are of course legal, but where some managers are grudging others are sympathetic. Sick leave of course is open to abuse, and if many episodes are taken either as prolonged leave or multiple short uncertificated breaks you may need to enquire in a more detailed way to find out what is going on. Not to do so is unfair to the person in question and to colleagues carrying the burden of their absence. There are some well-trodden paths to follow in such an enquiry.

For repeated short-term absences interview the employee to get her account of the reason. You may then need to refer the employee to the occupational health department if it seems that there is genuinely a chronic health problem. Beware however the multiple poorly explained absences that may represent alcohol problems. What you must *not* do when exploring reasons for absence is to start making clinical medical judgments about employees yourself, however tempting it may be. To be frank I think the convoluted business of "absence management", except perhaps where it applies to medical staff, is not the correct area for clinical managers to get into. It should be done by the personnel department with the assistance of your non-clinical manager.

Long-term sickness
Although this too should not be your business you are likely to be caught up in the process. Importantly you will need to remember your clinical habits of caring rather than your managerial reflexes that might view such absences as a drain on resources or just as a nuisance. Make sure that:

- Occupational health is involved.
- The employee is being contacted regularly at home.
- Reintegration plans are in place for the end of the illness.

If the ill health is such that premature retirement is needed, or worse that the employment must be terminated, you *must* contact your personnel officer to find out how to go through these processes. They are complex and need to be handled with the utmost sensitivity. In the rare and unhappy event of serious or terminal illness in one of your employees, you may need to chivy to make sure that the complex bureaucracy that surrounds early retirement on grounds of ill health works speedily and humanely.

Maternity leave
Remember that maternity leave is not funded from your clinical budget, so the problems for you are only to do with the appointment

of locums or the making of other arrangements. Do this early. The time when the mother to be leaves the organisation should be very predictable! Long locums in these situations are not too difficult to find but try to allow a handover period. Maternity leave is not necessarily paid leave and the necessary arrangements should be made through the personnel department. In some organisations paternity leave is acceptable though for much less time. Fathers intending to take such leave really must be encouraged to declare it early and the rules governing it within the organisation must be very explicit if it is not to degenerate into episodic uncovered absences. Returning from maternity leave may be a daunting prospect for many mothers who in prospect thought it would be straightforward but whose new postpartum, softer psyche sees the prospect of separation from her baby as nearly intolerable. Try to help by ensuring that someone keeps in touch with her while she is away and help her ensure that if she wishes to return, the proper creche or nursery arrangements have been made. Once she is back you will need to be sympathetic to her occasional need to arrive late or leave early or even be absent if her baby is sick.

Too much leave

A sensitive measure of a team's performance is sickness levels. While you should be of course sympathetic to genuine sick leave, you need to take a hard look at the reasons for multiple leave. Find out what sort of sick leave has been taken, is it one area or ward? How does it compare with other areas of the hospital? Does it have the features of inappropriate leave, for example Fridays and Mondays, during school holidays, during prebooked annual leave, when a particular manager or ward sister is on duty, or is it during major sporting events? Any of these enquiries can point to a managerial problem. These absences may not be just laziness but are often due to features such as undermanning leading to stress or to a confrontational style of leadership from a manager or ward sister. Try to correct that and if an individual is at fault, once again contact the personnel department, particularly if you think formal disciplinary processes are needed as these must be done "by the book".

4.1.2 Shrinking the team

It may be that for whatever reason you conclude that someone in your team has got to go, be fired, outplaced, relocated, made redundant, persuaded to retire, anything! In these circumstances, and as soon as that little spark comes into your head telling you that this is the solution, *do nothing, write nothing, say nothing.* Go immediately and confess to your personnel manager, because if the processes are not undergone in exactly correct detail you could find yourself in a seemingly endless spiral of appeals and tribunals that will make you wish you had never embarked on the process in the first place.

Concerning redundancy

It seems extraordinary that a few years ago mechanisms were established in London (and other big cities) to cope with what were expected to be a tide of redundancies of all grades following on from implementation of the mergers and bed reductions recommended in the Tomlinson Report. Now that we see a truer picture of what resources we need, we realise that we are in fact rather short of many staff, especially doctors and nurses, so it is rare that you will be making people redundant. If staff are made redundant there may be "slotting in" arrangements to enable them, for better or worse, to be accommodated in vacancies elsewhere in the organisation. If for any reason you have to make consultants redundant remember that it is prohibitively expensive to make anyone between 50 and 60 redundant (often the very person you might wish to be shot of). For the over sixties a negotiated early retirement is often a reasonable avenue to explore, but only after careful costing of the options by the personnel and finance departments.

4.2 Building a team

Managers and successful clinicians are only successful if they are part of a team. There are many teams within a hospital—the board, the executive, clinical directorates and smaller teams got together for specific purposes. The physiology and pathology of such teams is a large topic outside the scope of this book, but theory abounds and could hypothetically be used to build the perfectly effective and harmonious team.[1] Unfortunately, in most circumstances in the Health Service one's options about who can be recruited onto a team are limited. Indeed, as a medical manager recently appointed you will usually come to a basic preformed team, for example, a clinical services manager, a finance manager, someone from nursing, and someone from personnel. In that sort of team at least the members are already committed to the team's purpose; more worrying are teams that come together in the guise of committees where the tendency is for the team to be you and your managerial helper plus one consultant, one nurse, one junior doctor, one GP, all recruited by somebody else from a skimpy supply of volunteers.

If you do have the opportunity to put together a team yourself you should therefore:

(A) *Recruit from other than volunteers.* This may require some assiduous persuading of the "right" people. If you allow yourself to be victim of a pseudo-democratic process that simply delivers representatives to your team you may not get the skills or the commitment that you need, you may even get the opposite.

(B) Try to get *a functional mix of personality types.* You will, of course, make straightforward human judgments about this, but knowledge of Belbin types might help you achieve the right mix.[2] A brief summary of the Belbin types is given below:

   (1) *A Chairperson* presides over the team and coordinates its efforts to meet external goals and targets. He is distinguished by a preoccupation with objectives, sets the agenda and establishes priorities.

   (2) *The Shaper.* Just as the chairperson is the social leader, so the shaper is the task leader supplying a lot of personal input to shape the application of the team's efforts.

   (3) *The Plant* is the ideas person who tends to be original and radically minded; usually the most intelligent and imaginative member of the team.

   (4) *The Monitor/Evaluator.* This is the person who analyses and criticises the ideas that the team is working with and is good at assessing large volumes of data and analysing them objectively.

   (5) *The Company Worker* is the practical organiser who takes the decisions and strategies of the group and turns them into defined and manageable tasks that people can actually get on with.

   (6) *The Resource Investigator* is the member of the team who most easily goes outside the group to bring in new ideas; a social, gregarious team member but not a generator of original ideas.

(7)   *The Team Worker* is the member most sensitive to the psychology of the remainder of the team; a good listener and communicator who promotes unity and harmony in the team and works to avoid confrontation.

(8)   *The Finisher* is preoccupied with order, neatness and the completion of tasks.

It is hardly surprising that each of these characters has their own psychological type, and after many years of research Belbin was able to categorise them on the basis of their intelligence, dominance, extroversion/introversion and stability/anxiety scores.

The crucial members too often missing tend to be one of two types. Firstly *chairman/coordinator*, who sets the work of the team underway and structures that work (this should be you!). Secondly, you will find too few *finishers*; these characters are often self-effacing and quiet, not advertising themselves as potential members of the team.

(C)   *Define the overall tasks* of the team and of its individuals. These tasks should be SMART:

● Structured
● Measurable
● Achievable
● Realistic
● Timed.

In groups such as a hospital executive or a clinical directorate the tasks of a team are multiple and self-evident, but a formal exercise to identify them is nevertheless necessary, and in doing so it is also crucial to define the individual roles of the specific members of the team.

Having got the team together and defined its tasks, how do we make it work well? It is sometimes assumed that the common ideological goal of caring for patients is enough on its own to bond and motivate a multidisciplinary team, so perhaps it is not surprising how rarely anyone perceives the specific need to bond a team. All teams take time to establish themselves, members need to discover each others' personalities, work out their interpersonal difficulties, and define the group dynamics. Shared time and shared responsibilities will push a team together in due course and the clinical signs will be the appearance of "in jokes" and generally recognised alliances and tensions. The early stages of team development need some supervision, particularly where members of the team are seen regularly to be departing from the joint goals of the team. Such departures should be openly aired in the group if the disruptive members are not to be left regularly disrupting business. In achieving that it is of course crucial that the team should have a clear mandate and corporate perspective.

"Away days" are good bonding mechanisms as long as they are planned well ahead to allow clinicians to escape from their clinical work with a good conscience. "Away days" encompass the normal bonding activities of eating and drinking together, but fortunately within the Health Service we have not yet embraced the more extreme versions of this bonding activity where the team goes away to climb impossibly high mountains and swim in horribly cold lochs. I believe the evidence that such "outward bound" activities do much good is slim.

Similarly I have never discovered whether there is any evidence as to whether inclusion of partners (husbands, wives, *et al.*) at team social occasions is beneficial or disruptive. Partners must at a distance suffer many of the unpleasant side effects of the management process; the late arrivals, the early departures, the fallen soufflé, and the missed children's parties, so they may have little sympathy for it; but they also develop a sense of curiosity about the characters that people their partners' working lives. In my experience one of the difficulties with including partners is that most management teams have a good proportion of domestically dysfunctional members, such that the inclusion of partners in any team-building activities is out of the question.

Time is in short supply in the NHS, so once you have a satisfactory team delegation becomes crucial. Of course, the delegatees must understand what is expected of them over what timescale; feedback to them must be predictable and, when appropriate, congratulatory. There is a tendency in the Health Service for it to be believed that people will do the job for its own intrinsic worth and do not require the simple reward of recognition and congratulation.

4.2.1 Recruitment and appointment

As a medical manager one of your most specific tasks will be to do with recruitment and appointment and this will particularly affect you when it concerns consultants, senior nursing and managerial posts.

Recruitment

Doctors familiar with the career structure for doctors, and mindful perhaps of their own difficulties in getting the job they wanted, may assume that recruitment simply means advertising and waiting for the replies. Often it does, but there are now clinical areas, particularly psychiatry, anaesthetics, paediatrics, A&E and orthopaedics, where recruitment is difficult. A survey by the National Association of Health Authorities and Trusts in 1995 found that 79% of trusts had recruitment problems. The main reasons given for this were:

- Inadequate national work force planning.
- High drop-out rate among trainees.
- Inappropriate limitations on some consultant-grade posts.
- Inflexibility and delay in granting work permits for overseas doctors.[3]

The same study also found that 83% of trusts had had difficulty in recruiting in training grades in the same specialties mentioned above but also in general medicine and in elderly care. Difficulties in recruiting doctors can occur even in the most prestigious of organisations. If your hospital is not blessed by a good reputation and a nice address this may be a major issue for you and successful recruitment may even require you to change the job plan, the terms and conditions of service, or both. Even with extra effort put into recruitment, including recruitment overseas, you may still be unable to recruit and you may have to look at other ways of having the work done. In nursing the problem is worse and more worrying than it is for doctors. While you are unlikely to be involved in the day-to-day practical chores of appointing nurses because their turnover rate is so high that it is a full-time job, you will not escape having to deal with the consequences of the difficulty in recruitment. You will need to understand why this is more than a temporary problem and why simply increasing the effort to recruit may not be the long-term solution. Some simple facts and a basic knowledge of mathematics will suffice!

- 25% of all nurses will reach retirement age within the next 10 years. Less than 20% of registered nurses are under 30.

103

- Currently 20 000 new nurses are needed per year, by 2010 this will have risen to 25 000.
- Recruitment to nursing has fallen by 39% since 1988, currently only 16 000 per year enter nurse training.
- The private sector employed 30 000 nurses in 1990, 50 000 in 1995.
- The dropout rate from nurse training is 15–18%.
- New nursing roles outside original established positions are steadily being created.
- Nursing salaries consistently fall behind those of equivalent occupations outside the Health Service.
- The number of school leavers is falling.

There are in theory solutions and these are apparent from other data. There are 140 000 nurses currently not working and 69% of these claim that inflexibility of working hours is the major reason. In a recent Royal College of Nursing Survey 43% of all nurses claimed to have dependent children. While this is unsurprising, it does mean that to bring these nurses back into the workforce you will need to pay considerable attention and devote some of your budget perhaps to the provision of creche facilities and to the reorganisation of the pattern of working and the cultural attitudes to part-time work.

These solutions may also be applicable to the difficulties in recruiting doctors. Currently around 50% of medical graduates are female and the "wastage" rate is high largely because traditional forms of working and of training are incompatible with family life for those who have children. Even if medical mothers wish to return to work in due course, the system is unhelpful or even frankly obstructive. Those that stay on or come back tend to do so in general practice rather than in hospital practice.

For female doctors the problems are not just to do with child care facilities. They are also to do with part-time training and part-time working. We are very bad about facilitating this, especially in hospitals. HM (69)6 made provision for flexible training schemes for doctors, but even now only 7% of SpR posts are flexible and 2% of SHOs.[4] Hospitals are unenthusiastic about taking on these trainees and there are problems with funding. Such part-time training also seems to be unpopular with trainees, quite simply because most are half-time and thus only half the necessary training is achieved per year so the training needs twice as long.

The unpalatability of this leads to a number of trainees having incomplete training. Such doctors can only be fitted into non-consultant-grade posts. Unfortunately the abject resistance of the BMA to the establishment of meaningful non-consultant-grade posts has penalised people looking for part-time posts and the occupants of the posts are not a happy group. Over 50% of associate specialists are required to be involved in junior on-call rotas and few find that there are opportunities or funding for further education; almost all feel exploited. Even the term "non-career" grade has become a pejorative one, as if these doctors' commitment was less than total. As a medical manager, even without the BMA's support, there is plenty of leeway within the current regulations to make arrangements which will attract high-quality doctors who might otherwise be lost to the system, although you will almost certainly first have to do battle with the full-timers who tend to be unsympathetic.

If you have difficulty recruiting into normal full-time house officer and SpR posts you will need to review your unit's current performance against a well-recognised list of factors which discourage trainees from looking at certain jobs.[5]

- Insufficient supervision and support.
- Inadequate time and funding for study.
- Poor working environment, especially bad accommodation, and inadequate provision for meals out of hours.
- Absent processes for monitoring and responding to junior doctors' concerns.
- Failure to meet New Deal hours standards

The same sort of issues will of course affect the recruitment of nurses and others. You can as a manager in theory act to correct problems, but I have to admit that I am not alone in having had frustrating experiences of trying to persuade managers with no experience of front line working that abolishing or failing to maintain doctors' and nurses' residences and of making puny financial savings by abolishing proper eating facilities at night is counterproductive.

The process of appointing staff

For the purposes of this chapter let us fix on the appointment of consultants because it will be a certain role for the clinician in

105

management and because it is the type of appointment most beset by regulations. The process, however, has much in common with that for other senior appointments with which you might be involved.

Let's take the process step by step.

1. A vacancy is due

In general it is clear when a vacancy is due as most are consequent upon retirement. For a consultant appointment you really ought to begin the replacement process a year before the date of retirement. This is made difficult by consultants taking early retirement and being hesitant about the exact date. The first and often ignored step is openly to ask two questions:

- Do we really need to refill this post?
- If so, should it be the same job?

A retirement is a God-sent opportunity for change not to be wasted. If however after reflection a replacement is judged feasible, desirable and is funded, then you will need to concoct three documents. A job description, a job plan, and a person specification.

(a) Job description Much of this will follow a standard format (Table 4.1). The personnel department will usually write this with you, as most of the items are to do with such things as health clearance, patient confidentiality, leave, etc.

(b) Job plan It is important that this, like the job description, is tightly drawn. "Drift" used to be a real problem with consultant appointments. You would appoint someone to a post as a consultant geriatrician only to find him doing interventional endoscopy, or appoint a hand surgeon to discover that no hand service had been set up but breast reconstructions were on the increase! The job plan should specify the fixed sessions in detail. These are of course open to subsequent change but only by negotiation and agreement. The regional college or faculty advisor needs to ensure that it is properly balanced. The advisor has 3 weeks in which to comment, after that approval is assumed.

106

Table 4.1   Outline of the job description required for a consultant

Title of post	
Employing authority	
Place of employment	
Nature of appointment and hours of work	This explains that part-time employment is allowable
Background	This should give a snapshot of the hospital or unit and the team which the appointee will join
Overall purpose of the post	This must be very explicit and say what service the post-holder is to provide. To confirm that there is an emergency on-call rota and that cover is needed for absent colleagues on sick, annual and study leave. That the post-holder will need to undertake teaching and to participate in administration. That the post-holder will be committed to audit and to service development
Duties and responsibilities	This enumerates the number of sessions and lays out in detail where those sessions might need to be carried out
Firm structure and support services	This will enumerate the other members of the team, secretarial support, etc.
Managerial	This should outline the management structure of the unit in which the appointee will work
Health and safety	Points out the need for safe working, care of personal health and safety and includes specifics about attendance at occupational health, for instance to check hepatitis status
Confidentiality	Outlines the organisation's duty of confidentiality to patients and might usefully add a section on an individual's right to draw attention to deficiencies in the service
Timetable	This is the job plan
Terms and conditions of service	This may point out that Whitley Council provisions apply and outlines the annual leave allowance, equal opportunities regulations, superannuation, removal expenses, etc.

(c) The person specification You may have seen these for jobs outside medicine:

> The successful applicant will typically have 10 years' experience in worldwide dynamic marketing strategies, will be fluent in at least nine languages and have a persuasive and sunny disposition with nice white teeth—package 50–90K plus car, schooling, housing, profit-sharing scheme, and stupendously generous pension.

It is not like that in the NHS. Indeed you may feel that a person specification is superfluous. In spite of that it may help at least to draw up a basic matrix (Figure 4.1).

	Essential	Desirable
Qualifications		
Experience		
Skills		
Personal characteristics		

Figure 4.1   A basic matrix for a person specification.

There are of course dangers in these typed specifications; firstly you may get who you think you want rather than who you need and, secondly, you can become hostage to a team who have deliberately arranged a specification that excludes all but their preferred candidate. Whatever the specification it is important that the advertisement should not be too closely drawn and that the widest potential field of candidates is attracted.

2. Getting a short list

Once the post is advertised (it must be advertised) and a closing date and interview date are arranged, a list of those appropriate to select the candidate must be established. For consultant appointments this, and the remainder of the process, are carefully controlled by regulations. Short listing is carried out by the members of the Advisory Appointments Committee (AAC) and the interviewing is also, in theory, exclusively by the AAC. You should be familiar with the regulations that control these processes. They are explicit and readably set out in "The National Health Service (Appointment of Consultants) Regulations 1996. Good Practice Guidance". As new arrangements came into force on 1 April 1996 this guidance supersedes previous guidance. The AAC now consists of five core members. These will include one lay member, the chief executive or his deputy, the medical director or his deputy, a consultant normally from the relevant specialty and from the employing body and, lastly, a college-appointed assessor. The committee is required to have a majority of professional members and a majority of local members. University representatives will no longer be part of an AAC, except where the appointment is to a post which involves either substantial teaching or research commitments or both. If more than one trust or hospital is involved it is allowed to have extra members from the other organisation.

The local team and potential colleagues will have views about the candidates and will wish to arrange the right appointment. Those representing the hospital on an AAC may have a difficult line to tread in that they need to explore the views of the potential colleagues, even to the extent of having a formal meeting with them to discuss the CVs; but all must understand that no one can in advance bind AAC members to a particular choice. Candidates should be allowed the opportunity to visit the hospital and meet with potential colleagues; there may even be a joint meeting with consultants and the other candidates which they can attend. However, they do not have any obligation to attend such preinterview arrangements or "trials by cocktail party". Such gatherings are contentious and may be best avoided when planning appointments procedures. If there are such meetings care must be taken that questions are not asked of the candidates which would not be allowed in the formal interview. There should be additional wariness about the unvalidated prejudice that can be obtained through verbal references.

The dangers of unfairness in selection are manifold. Yet in our desire to be fair, give equal opportunities and be politically correct, we run the risk of blunting our powers to choose the right candidate. The sticklers for correctness have suggested, for example, that preinterview visits to the hospital should be forbidden and that all candidates must be asked the same questions at interview. Fortunately the AAC guidelines do not require that and allow us, for example, to ask "questions to ensure that candidates, men and women, married or single, can meet the requirements of the job, e.g. where it involves unsocial hours". Even so our means of selection are, to commercial organisations or hospitals in other countries, laughably rigid and inadequate. We do not test whether people might be able to work together, there is no psychological or specific aptitude testing or head hunting for elective appointments. The use of variations in salary to get the best candidate is almost unknown. Too much is left to the single, highly structured meeting of a single committee, often filled with people who have minimal experience of the field to which the appointment is being made. Such committees run the risk of appointing the glib, the personable and the paper-qualified candidate because of the shallowness of the assessment process.

References are largely worthless. They can confirm facts for the personnel department and check on absence record but because of the dangers of litigation few people are prepared to pass adverse comment, however honest. However, one must remember that failure to comment on known poor performance in a candidate risks the writer being brought before the GMC for professional misconduct. What is sometimes informative, if unintentionally so, is to see who the candidate has *not* cited for a reference; if it is the candidate's most recent boss, one needs to wonder why.

The role of college representatives is somewhat misunderstood. They are there to ensure the candidate is appropriately qualified, not to get the oldest, longest serving trainee on the rotation into the post.

It is interesting that although the members of an AAC are supposed to have equal opportunities training and be fluent in interviewing techniques, they have only rarely had any formal training to ensure in particular that:

- All candidates are allowed equal time to talk.
- Questions are "open".
- Each candidate is listened to for an equal length of time.
- The interview time for each candidate is the same.

Trained interviewers can achieve a 4 : 1 interviewer to interviewee talk time ratio, whereas for the untrained interviewer the average is 2 : 1, and for lay chairmen 1 : 1.[6]

A source of guidance on interviewing is the BMA's "Guidelines for Good Practice in the Recruitment and Selection of Doctors" (1994).

3. The appointment

When the AAC has made its recommendation, it is important to remember that it is just that. Indeed an AAC may make more than one recommendation. The actual appointment is made by the "employing authority", e.g. the board of the trust, though there would normally have to be exceptional reasons why an appointment was not confirmed and it only rarely happens. If the team within the hospital feels that the AAC has forced an inappropriate consultant on to them, they do at least have one last opportunity to make an appeal before ratification of the appointment. The employing authority can authorise one of its members, for example the chief executive or the medical director, to approve the appointment at the time of the AAC, but they can only do so if the AAC's recommendation is unanimous.

4. Induction

All staff joining a hospital should have a formal induction course, yet the Audit Commission assessment of trainees' hospitals showed that only 60% of all grades attend a general induction course for the hospital and only 30% attend one for their own specialty. For registrars these figures fall to 30% for a general course and 18% for a specific course. This is not the place to lay down the details of induction courses, but as a medical manager it is your responsibility to ensure that induction courses are in place and that the appropriate written material is available. A logical way to go about structuring an induction programme is to ask trainees who are leaving to say what it was they wish they had been told. In the absence of specific suggestions though proposed topics to cover on day 1 of induction programmes should be the following:

- Service processes and procedure (ordering investigations, hospital forms and notes, service departments, admitting and transferring procedures, discharge drugs, and procedures).
- Understanding hospital services (bleeps, switchboard, car parking, ID, support staff).
- Personal requirements (accommodation, house-keeping, catering facilities).
- Orientation to the new environment (mess and hospital facilities, meetings, timetables, rota).
- Essential practical skills (CPR, hospital computer, major disaster plan).
- Professional and financial concerns (P45, contracts, indemnity, rules relating to continuity of care, notification to coroner, liaison with GPs, etc.).
- Educational arrangements (identification of supervisor and tutor, sources of career advice, details of study leave).

That is a lot to cover in one day but it is possible, although a lot of young doctors complain of being completely punch drunk at the end of the induction day and of having remembered almost nothing! A newly appointed house officer is likely to be frightened and apprehensive, emotions not conducive to detailed learning!

111

4.3 Managing conflict

Hospitals are stressed and stressful places by the very nature of what they do. Staff feel passionately about the issues and have difficulty responding to change, to restrictions and to the under-provision of resources. Difficulty is made worse at a local level by the size and undemocratic structure of the NHS as a whole, which throws up a lot of "us against them" areas of conflict. Sadly there are also too many "us against us" issues to do with dominance, territory and power; the same sort of issues you would see in a colony of apes. Most NHS consultants have tasted battle too many times in these areas to be naive or easily outflanked. But these conflicts are the stuff of management.

The doctor involved in management is uniquely placed to handle conflicts within the organisation because his privilege is to hold formal power through office as a manager at the same time as having credibility as a clinician. Furthermore, he can get access to medical networks, can understand the clinical details of priorities and, crucially, can recognise clinical bullshit.

Donaldson[7] has summarised the sources of power in an organisation as:

- Holding formal authority.
- Controlling scarce resources.
- Having information.
- Possessing special expertise.
- Displaying the ability to cope with uncertainty.
- Commanding strong networks.
- Belonging to the dominant culture.

The medical manager qualifies in almost all of these categories. This does not, however, guarantee ease in reducing conflicts, but the following suggestions may be useful:

(1) *Be impartial.* If this is made impossible by your position, be ready to use an outside arbiter to validate facts presented by both sides in the conflict and confirm the options that are available for resolving it. The management consultant is often simply making money out of her independence rather than any special skill or knowledge of the problem.

(2) *Avoid win/lose situations.*

(3) *Keep the temperature down*, but make sure that all the players are informed of the facts of the issues. It is more difficult to retain a partisan position when the larger picture has been spelled out clearly.

(4) Sometimes it is necessary to *marginalise* one or more parties in a conflict. This should not be done in an aggressive sense but softly by exclusion from power areas or decision-taking bodies while leaving bridges open. This is not Machiavellian, it is simply pragmatic.

(5) *Avoid trade-offs*. While some trade-offs are inevitable in a negotiated solution to a conflict, try to avoid "buying-off" conflict if you can. Do not make promises of future goodies which you may not be able to deliver or worse which your successor will be expected to deliver.

(6) *Involve other members* of the team in the decisions that resolve the conflict.

(7) *Get the facts right*. Disputes often centre on a disagreement about the facts—try to get the right facts from an independent source.

4.3.1 Special areas of conflict

Management versus the medical advisory committee
As a paid up medical manager your relationship with the medical advisory committee in your hospital may be fraught. The medical advisory committee, or whatever it is called in your hospital, is not just a parliament of consultants getting together disinterestedly to advise the management, they are, by contrast, the historical rump of the old consensus management process of the 1970s and 1980s and still expect to have power. Insofar as their membership contains the consultants they have great power and no manager should forget it, but they also have a potential for great harm if allowed to fall prey to some of the archaic reflexes that such bodies can exhibit. The medical advisory committee can be like the Freudian Id, the dreaming subconscious, the expression of inappropriate, infantile wishes in a disorganised way that can seem meaningful to themselves though not to others; or if your prefer a different psychological allusion, they can tend to display irrational Dionysian thought rather than rational Apollonian thought. Whether or not medical advisory committees are constructive and helpful is, of

course, in their own hands. However bizarre their behaviour may sometimes be, the management side should never ignore it and should make every effort to ensure that the medical advisory committee is well informed, ideally in writing and in advance about what the organisation is up to, including the facts on which decisions of the management side of the organisation are based (particularly financial data). There are arguments about whether a medical advisory committee should be chaired by someone who is party to the current management and board thinking, for it can be valuable for resolving conflicts. One hopes that as more and more doctors have had the experience of the management of healthcare polarisation between management and the medical advisory committee will become less of an issue.

Purchasers of healthcare

For hospital trusts the relationship between the medical manager and the purchasing authority and the public health doctors who work for/with them occurs at the collision point between one group within the NHS, the providers, who tend to feel that they should make the running in defining what services are needed and how those services should be organised, and another increasingly empowered group, the purchasers, who feel it is they who better understand what is needed and are the proper definers of how it is to be delivered. So it is hardly surprising that sparks sometimes fly in meetings (politely of course). The competitive, market-based reforms of the Thatcher era and the then recent splitting of purchasing from providing made many purchasers overbold in their dealings with providers. The public health doctors employed by the purchasing authorities and newly empowered by that did not always realise the weakness of their data and the wider ramifications of the flexing of their purchasing muscles. By contrast, the medical and service directors of hospitals were unsympathetic to needs for service rationalisations and the restrictions of an inadequate purchasing budget. As the players and the data on which decisions are made become more sophisticated one hopes that cooperation will be more evident, though no doubt practising clinicians will be forever suspicious of the views of those who are not actually engaged at the coalface. Whatever the context, medical managers will need to be aware of the potentially prickly nature of the relationship.

4.4 Contracts and job descriptions

Older doctors consider medicine to be a vocation as well as a profession, and as such it might be considered in need of only the most minimal of contracts and a job description in the form simply of an indicative timetable of fixed commitments. My consultant contract when I was appointed was an all-embracing six paragraph statement simply reminding me of my responsibility to work to the best of my abilities for the hospital and its patients. The policing of such contracts was left to the conscience, peer pressure, and the General Medical Council (GMC). Unfortunately there is a need to control the minority who abuse the spirit of such contracts and such contracts were, in addition, the product of a steady state and of no use to the manager afloat on a sea of continuous change. The downside of the unfortunate habit of bureaucratisation in the Health Service has however led to contracts becoming more verbose, more detailed, and perhaps less flexible. Contracts between doctors and their employers are now underpinned by a job plan which defines the "fixed sessions" that they are expected to work. The contracts themselves are primarily directive, identifying a doctor's responsibilities, but they also carry some reference to the facilities that the employer will provide for the doctor and the teams in which he will work. Additionally they outline the framework which governs both parties' options when a change in job plan is needed.

As a manager—medical or otherwise—it is difficult to see how the work of doctors can be monitored or changed without such a template against which to measure it, but the risks of the plan itself and a managerial obsession with it are legion. The primary problem is that the plan's very explicitness can be perceived as implicitly denying trust and loyalty. Nevertheless, though there was much resistance to job plans when first proposed they are now generally accepted and understood not as a weapon of coercion but as a map of what a doctor does and a starting point for planning the clinical service or for altering it. Their existence also allows a process of regular review.

The British Medical Association issues guidelines on the completion of job plans which are sensible and do not deny the need for such plans. It is thus a rash medical manager who tries to impose some new format of his own and most do not, although it is reasonable to build on the concept of accountability which the job plan implies and to add other features. Your own organisation will have its habits in this respect, but as an example Guy's & St Thomas' Trust requires its consultants not only to complete a job plan but also to send in a diary of leave and study leave and to account for how flexible sessions are being used. All this forms the basis for an annual review.

4.4.1 Annual review

The bureaucracy of management has an annual cycle to it; the financial year for setting and closing budgets, the medical staffing year revolving around the times of appointment for new staff, the business planning cycle rotating around what purchasers demand and, lastly, if you are a clinical director, you will need to fit into the cycle an annual review of job plans incorporating ideally, a performance review. You should be reviewing all staff. Managers (including you) are reviewed against the tasks that were set for them, trainee doctors against their educational targets, and consultants against their job plans.

4.4.2 Consultants' review

It is part of the habit of the autonomy that British consultants enjoy that they may experience emotional difficulty coming to terms with the notion of an annual review. Therefore, from the outset of the process you need to ensure that it is clear that the review is a two-way event occurring in an informal setting where you can both review the continuing appropriateness of the job plan, discover whether there are any skills which need sharpening and what the organisation can do to assist in this process. Unfortunately, most clinical directors have no access to a budget for study leave and professional development with which to back up the conclusions of the review, but at the very least the opportunity to review each consultant's contributions may help with the business planning process which follows it. Rightly or wrongly annual reviews seem rarely to be followed by significant change, but given the vagaries of the assessment process this may be sensible. Microsoft is said to grade its employees with marks 1 to 5; 4 means exceptional, 1 means you're out! The other fashionable review process is the 360° review where each employee is assessed by her superiors, her peers and her subordinates. It would be fascinating in the NHS, but fascination alone must be the wrong motive for introducing it.

Staff appraisal, i.e. review of personal qualities rather than an objective assessment of practical performance adherence to job plan, etc., is a more risky activity. If it is to be done it must of course be done very, very sensitively and by someone competent enough and senior enough to make the appraisal; I must however confess to sympathy with Courtis' view:[8]

> Staff appraisal is becoming more popular. Avoid it like the plague ... Good people take their merits for granted and sometimes don't want to know about their demerits. Average people can be demotivated by being reminded how average they are. Below average people can be hopelessly damaged by being told about faults which they do not have the brains or personality to surmount.

Those truths apart there are other pitfalls in the appraisal process with which the medical manager needs to be familiar:[9]

- Prejudice.
- Insufficient knowledge of the individual.
- The "halo" effect of general likeability or recent events.
- The difficulty in distinguishing the individual's performance from the context in which he works.
- Different perceptions of the standards required.
- Avoiding a difficult decision; everyone passes, no honours, no fails.
- Ignoring the outcome of the appraisal.

4.5 Rewards

It is normal to assume that everybody needs rewards if they are to function well and to be happy. There are a few joyless psychologists who say that, by contrast, reward demotivates or encourages jealousy and a sense of injustice. However that thesis does not stand up scientifically[10] and realistically we manage in a reward-driven environment. In the NHS we have rewards but they are a rum mix. Doctors have a sophisticated and generous financial reward system in the form of good salaries augmented by merit awards and that is in addition to the gratification they get from being top dogs. Managers get promotion, PRP or some equivalent and manual workers get a whole range of archaic supplements to their pay and the nurses get ... well sadly, the nurses get nothing much except public approval, though that might change in the next century if the concept of the "nurse consultant" gains ground. All of us get the rewards of working with and for people in a cooperative and worthy venture. It is a measure of the value of that ultimate job satisfaction that in spite of the erosion of the sense of belonging to an institution, in spite of the abuses of our time and patience by the worsening bureaucracy, in spite of the culture of complaint, most of us love what we do. Very little erodes the four prime rewards of being a professional—collegiality; respect; variety; responsibility.

Nevertheless, as medical managers we should not expect these to be the sole drivers of the workforce and we have an obligation to keep a regular eye on the rewards that staff get, how they get them and how best to build on them, or at worst how to prevent their erosion. As a medical manager you need to understand the detailed mechanics of the financial reward systems that exist for doctors, discretionary awards and merit awards.

4.5.1 Non-financial rewards

The capacity to reap the intrinsic rewards flowing from the exercise of compassion and the pleasure of doing a job well is something people bring with them to a job. It may be the greatest motivator of all and it is certainly the one applicants for admission to medical school cite. It is not in the gift of managers, but other non-financial rewards are, importantly:

(1) The setting of identifiable and achievable goals.
(2) Feedback to recognise achievement.
(3) The allocation of responsibility appropriate to the person so that they can use their abilities optimally.
(4) The facilitation of personal development and further education.

For some staff these things are already formalised. House officers for example have little booklets given to them on their first day explaining what their goals are. There are forms at the back of the booklet to be filled in jointly with the trainer, ensuring that they have met to discuss progress and to recognise achievement. Simple they may be, but popular for some reason they are not. The reasons for ignoring these structured systems of goal setting is one suspects largely laziness on the part of both players. For house officers, goal setting is a relatively straightforward task. For other staff it may be a more difficult business requiring assessment, not only of the tasks that they need to achieve, but also the "core competencies" needed to achieve these tasks. If these assessments are to be linked to financial reward, then one also needs a process for recognising extra effort beyond the basic task. It is important to remember, however, that research finds that financial reward is considered to be a surprisingly unimportant part of the motivation for most staff.

4.5.2 Financial rewards

In essence the NHS works on a system of "pay spines" with increments. The newly appointed SpR starts at a particular salary and moves up willy-nilly to the top. Extra hours are paid but no account is taken of her skills or the effort she puts in. There are no extrinsic incentives to perform well, though she will need to pass her exams to stay in the grade, and be tolerably competent, courteous and hard working if she is to get references to rise out of one pay spine and into the consultant pay spine. For managerial staff there are no exams and no major progression up the spine except by promotion. Managers may, however, be rewarded by PRP and, less commonly, by skill-based pay. The problem with both of these is in assessing achievement. PRP in essence is a system for defining goals prospectively, and then retrospectively measuring the employee's performance in achieving the goals. PRP can be used to define progress through incremental grades or as an end of the year bonus measure.

For the employer the difficulties are in setting the goals accurately and in a subsequent assessment, particularly when weighing achievement in adverse rather than favourable environments. For the employee, the rewards on offer may not justify the frustrations of achieving them, as 3–5% of salary is the usual sort of range for PRP and most will not get the full sum. PRP, though widespread, is a difficult area for medical managers to become involved in and perhaps best avoided.[11] A study of PRP in the public services undertaken by the London School of Economics concluded that it sours relationships, undermines morale, and encourages favouritism.

More popular are targeted rewards, either for groups or individuals. For example operating theatre staff may all get a one-

119

off, end-of-year bonus if throughput has increased, or staff may individually receive a payment if they have taken no more than a defined time off sick.

Discretionary points and merit awards

When the original merit award system was in place, doctors could receive C, B, A or A+ merit awards. These represented a pensionable salary uplift of 25%, 50%, 75% or 100% respectively. Originally, once awarded they were for the duration of the doctor's employment, now they are reviewed every 5 years, although it is extremely rare for them to be taken away.

The C merit award was replaced in 1996 by the discretionary points system.

Discretionary points

Discretionary points are awarded only after the consultant has achieved the maximum on the consultant salary scale. "They are paid at the discretion of the employer (i.e. the trust or health authority) in the light of professional advice." There are five points in the scale. Associate specialists and those with part-time and with honorary contracts are also eligible. Any number of points may be awarded to a consultant at one time but after an award of points a consultant should not normally be considered until 2 years have elapsed. The total number of points which a trust can award to its eligible consultants should not exceed the sum of 0.25 per eligible consultant. Eligible consultants are those who have reached the top of the incremental scale and who do not hold a B, A or A+ award.

The whole process is run locally and medical managers, especially the medical director, should be central to the process of awarding points. The business of awarding discretionary points and merit awards is invariably criticised (by the have-nots), and the process used must therefore be very open and the criteria for the awards plainly spelled out. The criteria which have been identified by the NHS Executive are shown in Table 4.2.

It is up to the local management to decide how to make the assessment, but a graded list from clinical managers is essential. A system of voting by the whole body of clinicians has a tendency to recognise the gregarious and the well-socialised to the detriment of the quiet lab. worker. Discretionary points are an improvement

Table 4.2   Guidelines on criteria for consultants' discretionary points

The following principles should underpin the local implementation of the scheme:

(1) Discretionary points are *not* seniority payments, nor automatic annual increments

(2) Consultants in all specialties and all types of post are equally eligible and should be treated as such

(3) To warrant payment of a discretionary point, consultants will be expected to demonstrate an above average contribution in respect of service to patients, teaching, research and the management and development of the service

(4) Progression at each step up the discretionary point scale will reflect the increasing quality and range of the contribution made by the consultant. To attain the maximum of the discretionary point scale consultants will be expected to have demonstrated an outstanding contribution to services

(5) The criteria for payment of discretionary points should allow for contributions made in the following areas to be taken into account:
    (i) professional excellence, including
        —quality of clinical care of patients
        —service development
        —professional leadership
        —improvements in public health
    (ii) contribution to professional and multidisciplinary teamworking
    (iii) research, innovation and improvement in the service
    (iv) clinical audit
    (v) administrative or NHS management contributions
    (vi) teaching and training, including
        —training of junior staff
        —involvement in undergraduate or postgraduate teaching
        —public education and health promotion
        —contribution to training of other staff
    (vii) wider contribution to the work of the NHS nationally

(6) The differing opportunities and normal expectations associated with consultants in different fields will need to be taken into account in assessing the level of performance required in individual cases. For example, there will be a different expectation in terms of the research content of many honorary contract holders compared with consultants whose duties result in limited opportunities for research work. There would similarly be a different expectation in terms of the management and services development contribution of a consultant in public health medicine or dental public health compared with more clinically based specialties

(7) The resources available to a consultant, including supporting staff and facilities, and any particular difficulties that he or she may have had to overcome, should also be taken into account in judging the service contribution expected and provided

(8) In deciding payments employing bodies should ensure that consultants are treated equally regardless of their colour, race, sex, religion, politics, marital status, sexual orientation, membership or non-membership of trade unions or associations, ethnic origin, age, or disability

on the all-or-none quality of C awards, as they allow a better spread of reward. It might be thought that the slow progress to full allocation of points would delay the chance of a B award, but

121

B awards are given for slightly different criteria and it is not necessary to have a full set of discretionary points before being considered for a B award.

Merit awards

The merit award scheme was revised in 1995 and the details of its mechanics and outcomes are clearly spelled out in Executive Letter (95)109 which should be read by any clinical manager involved in assessing colleagues for merit awards. Several important features can however be summarised here:

- There is a fixed number of awards—about 14% of consultants hold an award and by retirement 25% will hold an award.
- Part-time consultants are paid pro rata in relation to their sessional commitment.
- No awards are granted after the age of 62.
- Rewards are reviewed every 5 years or earlier if there are "misgivings" about the award holder.
- Those in full-time management posts are not eligible but their awards are protected and reapplied when they return to clinical practice.
- Consultants who are re-employed into a substantive post after retirement can continue to be paid their award but not if the re-employment is as a locum.
- Recommendations may be made by individual trusts, by professional bodies and indeed by individuals.
- There is an appeal system.
- A list of those who hold awards is made public.

To receive a B or A award clinicians would normally need to be nominated by their trust. Nowadays the management side of a trust has an input, so clinicians who abandon their NHS trust for the sake of a high-profile life of national or international activities are less likely than they were to be rewarded. It was not always so. I am aware of one consultant awarded a very high award for national work who at the same moment narrowly avoided disciplinary procedures within the trust because of poor attendance at fixed commitments. Such awards were doubly galling for trusts when the trust itself was responsible for paying the extra salary for largely absent clinicians. Things are better now. The emphasis in the future is to be placed more on honest hard work within the

NHS, less stress will be put on elitist activities outside the trust. Additionally, the fraction of the salary which is the merit award, is now paid centrally instead of being taken from the trust's normal budget.

Once the trust itself has decided on its nominees, a regional and then a national committee will process them before the final decision is made. The process takes about a year and is complex. There are many checks and balances within it and it is fairly immune from inappropriate nominations. This does not, however, prevent the ritual expressions of outrage appearing in the press each year when the awards are announced. Such outbursts were previously directed at the secrecy of the process, but more recently have been focused on a presumption of racial discrimination or sex discrimination or favouring certain specialties (for some curious reason nuclear medicine comes off best). This is good fodder for the purveyors of political correctness and for any politician who would wish to see an end to a system of merit awards, but it is rarely noted that such apparent inequalities are more a comment on the role played in the NHS by women and racial minorities than they are of the awards process itself. If women and ethnic minorities do not write papers and books or chair committees or get elected to the council for this or that or become professors, that is not the fault of the merit award process or the means by which we measure that merit. The Commission for Racial Equality looked at the scheme in 1997 and was unable to find evidence of discrimination at work within it.

It is probably safe to assume that the existence of a merit award system is a significant driver of consultant commitment to achievement over and above what is inherent in their daily work. Other systems of reward have been proposed to replace it, such as targets and rewards for clinical teams, as distinct from individuals. These do point up the importance of efficient team working and the need for mechanisms to encourage that, but they overlook the crucial importance of motivation working at a personal level. They also forget that many of the tasks in the NHS, especially those recognised by merit awards, are not team activities but individual ones.[12]

And in case you were wondering, as I suspect you were, whether medical management posts increase the chance of being awarded a merit award the answer at the moment has to be "Don't know". Clinicians in management are more likely than their peers to have a merit award, but whether that is related to their management activities is unknown. (J Simpson, Chief Executive BAMM, personal communication).

4.6 Problems with colleagues

One of the most intriguing effects of time spent in medical management is the exposure it gives you to the character of your colleagues. Not only colleagues in particular, but doctors in general. I found this unexpected, for I thought I knew my colleagues; indeed I did, but only as friends where they were friends or as professional colleagues whom I judged as professionals. Were they a good opinion? Were they nice to patients? Were they prompt and diligent when referred a patient? What was surprising was how poor a predictor these skills are of the different abilities doctors now need. For example, the ability to work in teams particularly when they are not the boss (the jargon phrase, I believe, is "cooperating in flatter, non-hierarchical structures"). Also, their ability to handle change. In the face of change some of the nicest and best doctors expose themselves as the most abject reactionaries, blind to reason and prone to prima donna tantrums and the wilful misuse of facts. I don't know what percentage of clinicians fall into this category, but one analysis of a non-medical organisation noted that 10% were "eagles" (leaders), 80% "sheep" (passively led), and 10% "mules" (obstructivist). I think the mule quota is a low estimate for clinicians, though I hope we also have more eagles.

Problems with colleagues fall into four distinct categories:

(1) *The difficult colleague.* Clinically competent, fine with patients and staff but often intransigent and uncooperative with managers and any others who try to control this colleague.
(2) *The naughty/improper colleague.* Clinically competent but rude and offensive to colleagues and patients, or whose timekeeping is unsatisfactory. These may be frank breaches of the trust's disciplinary regulations or may fall short of disciplinary error.
(3) *The incompetent and/or dangerous colleague.* This group is dealt with in Section 4.6.3.
(4) *The sick colleague.* Sick doctors are discussed in Section 4.8.

4.6.1 The difficult colleague

Difficult colleagues are numerically only a small part of the workforce, but they are a real problem because they consume

124

an inordinate amount of a medical manager's time and energy. Unfortunately you do not have a formula for dealing with them as you do with the doctor who is incompetent or breaks the rules. Furthermore, the obstructive colleagues are the very ones who are least likely to accept your right as a medical manager to ask for changes in the way they practice, and they certainly will not have any sympathy for your occasional need to pass comment on the way they conduct their personal clinical practice. If they are rabble-rousers and busy letter writers they become more than a nuisance and are often frankly damaging. Management books and courses are replete with advice on how to deal with this sort of person in an organisation, the "squeaky wheel", but in any particular instance the advice, like so much in management books, differs little from common sense. They will also recount the psychological personality types and parade for you a gallery of quirky personalities that can cause trouble. These certainly raise a smile when you recognise among them the obdurate, obstructive bastard who is causing you so much trouble, but they rarely tell you *how* to deal with him. You may however, find the "transactional analysis" view of inter-personal relationships helpful.[13] This looks at the kind of interaction you may have with your difficult colleague. Each of you in any particular contact is acting either as a parent or a child or an adult. Transactions can be:

- *Complementary.* Such as natural, e.g. parent–child or adult–adult.
- *Crossed.* Where the opening approach receives an inappropriate response; e.g. manager: "can we discuss how we are going to deal with the waiting list?" (*adult*), clinician: "no, I'm too busy and it's your problem not mine" (*child*).
- *Ulterior.* These are more complex but the commonest is exemplified by the real message being disguised under an explicit socially acceptable message.

Transactional analysis stresses the importance of looking at the *feelings* that generate the heat in transactions that are seemingly about *facts*.

Of course, you should in the correct parental, adult way try to explain and persuade, but I have to conclude that to protect yourself and the other work that needs to be done, obdurate mules are often best managed by being simply marginalised, and the river of events merely allowed to flow on around them. There are, however, some basic principles to apply in your dealings with obdurate colleagues:

(1) Listen courteously and open mindedly.
(2) Do not allow your replies to be aggressive or threatening. Somebody with a grievance is more of a problem than somebody who is simply a nuisance.
(3) Leave bridges open for late conversion.
(4) Do not get involved in protracted exchanges of letters.
(5) Make sure your policy is shared with your managerial colleagues to avoid the obdurate clinician simply trying to bypass you.
(6) Always refute quietly but publicly attempts to raise the temperature by the use of false data.
(7) Try to explain the broader picture. The obdurate clinician is usually more concerned about small and personal issues and hasn't, can't or won't see the broader picture.

In these matters most of one's colleagues are supportive and understand the issues, and therefore one should not let them down by taking the easy option of giving in to the noisy one.

4.6.2 The naughty/improper colleague

Doctors get away with a lot that they should not. Latitude in personal attendance and behaviour has often been tolerated out of an archaic subservience to an imagined professional ethos that protects and insulates the doctor from the work-a-day world. Bad behaviour such as rudeness is often tolerated in doctors as a charming quirk of character—the Sir Lancelot Spratt phenomenon; charming quirks of character which, when exhibited by a porter, lead promptly to his dismissal.

The social culture in which we work has changed and while quirkiness itself may lend colour to a drab world, quirkiness that is naughtiness or impropriety needs to be changed. No one is better placed to do this than the clinician in management. The recurring problems which he will have to deal with are non-attendance and late attendance at fixed commitments, rudeness to patients and staff, and denigration or harassment of other staff. In my experience the difficulty in these situations is getting the problem in proportion and not over- or under-reacting. Your non-involved

colleagues will be watching very closely. The following suggestions
may be useful:

(1) Get the facts right. If there is an allegation of rudeness or
     harassment get the facts from the victim in writing. People
     are often unwilling to do this, but without something solid to
     back you up you are unlikely to make much impact on the
     malefactor who simply denies it all. The victim may not be
     prepared to put it in writing but you do at least need to get
     a promise that she will speak about the issues in front of
     you with a witness present. If possible, it is wise to obtain
     corroboration. Is it just one person who finds the doctor
     difficult or offensive or is it a shared perception among the
     team? Is the event about which the complaint is made merely
     an opportunity to convert a longstanding grudge into punitive
     action?

(2) Having decided to go ahead deal with the matter firmly. The
     first conversation need not be formal but subsequent ones
     should be.

(3) Remember that any formal meeting to discuss a problem
     should be documented (I send a letter afterwards summarising
     what was said). Try to have a colleague manager with you
     and offer the clinician a chance to bring someone with them.

(4) Always try for an informal resolution. Formal procedures
     are protracted, time consuming, painful and sometimes even
     counter-productive, and at the very least they are a distraction.

(5) Occasionally the complainant will agree that help is needed
     to improve his attitude, although this is rare. There are no
     equivalent of Maoist re-education camps available in the
     Health Service; what's needed is a network of trained,
     sympathetic clinicians and/or psychologists and/or medical
     directors, such that a colleague who wants help can be referred
     outside the organisation for that help. Unfortunately, to my
     knowledge, no such formal network exists; certainly none is
     known to the Association of Trust Medical Directors.

In this section I have not outlined a sequence of formal
disciplinary procedures. Although these tend to be much the same
from trust to trust, they often differ in detail and it is important
that the medical manager reads her own trust's disciplinary
procedures very carefully prior to instigating any formal action

against a colleague. We are all familiar with the fictional policeman who fails to achieve the true guilty verdict on a criminal simply because he neglected to act "by the book" or read the suspect his "rights". Formal hearings in the medical context should also be done by the book, so you ought to have read the book! Don't expect the regulations about disciplinary proceedings to be easy reading, and in general it is advisable to consult your director of personnel about the practicalities before acting. The Association of Trust Medical Directors has produced a useful practical document about this.[14]

If you are in a position where a disciplinary process becomes necessary, the "Hot Stove" principle of Macgregor is a useful *aide-mémoire* to ensure your evenhandedness and consistency. Douglas Macgregor was an American industrial psychologist who likened the well-tailored disciplinary process to touching a red hot stove:[15]

- The burn is immediate, so there is no question of cause and effect.
- There was a warning: the stove was red hot, and you knew what would happen if you touched it.
- It is consistent: everyone who touches the stove gets burned.
- It is impersonal: you get a burn not because of who you are but because of what you've done.

Political correctness issues

Formal complaints about the staff behaving in a "politically incorrect" way seem rare, but they are potentially difficult to deal with. Doctors often behave in a "politically incorrect" but well-meaning way. The normal banter between male doctors and female nurses is long established but potentially misinterpretable in the current climate. Many doctors find the linguistic fascism of the new correctness both ludicrous and unhelpful, and this may make potential trouble for the medical manager who may not understand the passion which some people attach to political correctness. An event which may seem to you to be absurdly trivial but which is perceived by someone on the staff as a major injustice may trip you up, and the humourlessness of the victim culture that underlies the political correctness movement may depress and irritate you. Nevertheless, mixed in with these irritations are true injustices that need acting upon.

The commonest way in which PC issues come up are:

(1) As alleged harassment, usually racial or sexual.
(2) As attempts to make you change language or procedures to be PC.

The process for dealing with the former should be straightforward in that it should not differ from any other disciplinary process and your trust's disciplinary rules should explicitly include harassment. The difficulty is where harassment is perceived but not intended—where politically incorrect speech for instance is perceived as harassment. This may afford you the opportunity for some difficult tight-rope walking, particularly at present where many disciplinary procedures, themselves couched in PC language, state that harassment exists if a person believes themselves to be harassed.

4.6.3 The incompetent colleague

We know that doctors are not perfect and the clinical skills and human relations of many are suboptimal. We know that medicine deals at its core with the fallibility of humans and that doctors are no different from other humans, but nevertheless a small number are simply so bad as to be dangerous. If the quality of medical care is to improve and if doctors are to be safer we need to have processes in place to identify and then improve or remove dangerous doctors and to improve the standard of the safe but poorly performing doctor.

A sequence of milestones must be passed before these objectives can be achieved:

(1) *Insight*. Doctors need sufficient insight to understand that they need continuous refreshing and re-education. This dimension is too often missing, although the evidence suggests that the prevalence of audit meetings and the habit of peer group review is gradually eroding this misplaced confidence. Doctors also need insight into their own illnesses and their ways of dealing with their own illnesses, something they tend to do badly through an innate perception that "doctors don't get ill".[16]
(2) *Identification*. An awareness that if others are repeatedly

129

clinically risky then one does not just look away. All clinicians have a duty to protect patients. Doctors who are quick to point out the dangers of an under-funded Health Service are sometimes slow to act to do anything about a fully funded but incompetent colleague.

The process of identifying and trying to help inappropriate performing doctors and their patients is a contentious one and has led to the much debated "shop-a-doc" legislation discussed below.

(3) *Re-training.* Once poor performers are identified by themselves or others in a hospital setting re-training options must be available if needed and support must be provided for the aged or ailing doctor. If the problem is illness, whether psychiatric, drug induced, alcoholic or whatever, the support is needed for that too (see Section 4.8). A more difficult situation is where the doctor fails to understand she is performing badly and rejects advice. A more formal process is then needed to protect patients.

(4) *Professional review.* Only if internal hospital processes fail or for some reason are impossible will the problem need to be passed to the General Medical Council (GMC) for its professional review process. It should be noted that even if hospital internal processes are underway or successfully completed, reports about malperforming doctors may reach the GMC by other routes, for example the public or the community health council. In relation to the GMC it is important to remember that poor performance is not about a single episode, it is about consistent or repeated failures, and it is about the performance of clinical tasks. It must never be a way of resolving internal trust wrangles about disciplinary matters such as late attendance.

When dealing with defects of performance whether internally or using the GMC care must be taken to confirm that the defects are real and documentable. It is not sufficient for a cabal of doctors and managers to take against a clinician because he is inept or lazy or not to their taste and then expect the GMC to resolve the problem for them.

The intention of the GMC process is remedial not disciplinary. However, if the investigation turns up information which suggests that disciplinary procedures are needed by the trust then the GMC will trigger those processes.

For details of the GMC professional review processes see below.

In all disciplinary and performance enquiries remember:

- Get the facts right.
- Act promptly.
- Act openly.
- Keep records.
- Do not take sides.
- Take advice from the personnel department.
- Remember the objective is the protection of patients.

"Shop-a-doc."

A lot of heat has been generated by the debate about doctors telling someone about colleagues who are performing poorly. Note that I have used the phrase "telling someone about". That does not sound too threatening. If I had written "informing on colleagues" who are performing poorly hackles would rise, but perhaps only for semantic reasons; "inform on" smacks of Eastern Europe or war-time collaborators. The reflex not to "sneak" on a colleague to someone in authority is deep rooted in the English psyche. E. M. Forster is famously quoted as saying he hoped he would have the courage to betray his country rather than a friend. The "shop-a-doc." fuss is more subtle. It arises from attempts following the Health Department 1995 report "Maintaining Medical Excellence" to enshrine in doctors' contracts an obligation to report poorly performing colleagues. Quite reasonably the BMA and others objected to this, pointing out that it was an ethical not a contractual issue. One hopes that no one quibbles with the ethical principle. The GMC rules are quite explicit on this, and indeed in the folder which contains each doctor's annual registration certificate there is a list of duties for doctors, one of which clearly states "act quickly to protect patients from risk if you have good reason to believe that you or a colleague may not be fit to practice". A BMA survey in 1995 showed that 88% of 814 respondants would be willing to act "if a colleague was failing to meet appropriate medical standards".[17] Following on from this the Central Consultants and Specialists Committee (CCSC) of the BMA issued guidance in October 1997 which requests consultants informally to deal with problems perceived in colleagues but notes that if that is unsuccessful "the doctor's duty must be to bring the matter formally to the attention of the Trust or other employer". The guidelines also stress the particular responsibility of clinical directors and medical directors to acknowledge and to act on concerns transmitted to them.

The issue then is that dangerous doctors need to be identified whatever your queasiness about the process. But how do we disentangle gossip from reality and protect patients while being fair to colleagues? The answer lies in a clear and accepted process. This is more likely to succeed if led by doctors, so they have the responsibility to establish, communicate and police the policy. Traditionally, medical advisory committees like to do this separately from the hospital administration, and the process of the "three wise men" existed to deal with part of the problem in relation to sick doctors. Nevertheless, in the current situation where there are many doctors in management it is neither appropriate nor necessary for medical advisory committees to keep these issues "in house"; clinical directors and/or the medical director must always be informed that a process is underway even if the medical advisory committee and its officers are to be the prime movers. There are those who object to this, but they should remember that a trust carries both legal and moral responsibilities for its patients as well as bearing the financial risks of medical negligence. If a group of clinicians take upon themselves the responsibility for deciding about inept colleagues and to do so without the knowledge and cooperation of the trust, they put themselves personally in a difficult position if a disaster occurs.

4.7 General Medical Council procedures for the assessment of poor performance (by Brian Ayers, Medical Director, Guy's and St Thomas' Hospital Trust)

The GMC logo is "Protecting patients, guiding doctors". These two principles are maintained through the introduction of performance assessment.

It is as well to remind ourselves of the background to these new procedures by remembering that the GMC was created under a Medical Act of Parliament in 1858 specifically to improve medical education and to set standards of practice. It exists to protect the public interest and the good name of the profession. The GMC is made up of 54 doctors elected by the profession, 25 doctors appointed by university medical schools and postgraduate institutions, and 25 lay people who are nominated by the Privy

Council. In recent years the number and influence of the lay membership has increased. The GMC is an independent statutory body and is not a government agency, not part of the NHS, not involved in organising or providing healthcare, not an employer of the medical workforce in this country, nor is it the doctors' union.

The new performance procedures come under the Fitness to Practise Division, which was created in 1858 to deal with serious professional misconduct and convictions. In 1980 a further Act was passed through parliament to deal with health issues of doctors which were sufficiently serious to impair fitness to practise. The performance procedures have been introduced to deal with seriously deficient performance. It should be noted that these three only deal with serious situations. The GMC is not involved in dealing with variations of practice which do not threaten the patient or public.

Within the Fitness to Practise Division there is an organisation for screening all complaints that are received. The screeners are members of the GMC who are given specific training to make discreet enquiries to identify whether there is a prima facie case requiring further investigation. If the screener decides there is concern, then health issues take precedence over conduct issues over performance issues.

The health procedures are private and confidential and aimed to be remedial. If the doctor cooperates the matter can be handled entirely locally and assessment is based on the opinion of medical experts.

Conduct procedures on the other hand are formal, public and adversarial. They are designed to deal with specific incidents, but do not allow the GMC to investigate a doctor's general standard of practice. There are no provisions for formal counselling, re-training or re-assessment where there is evidence of poor performance. Therefore, the conduct procedures can investigate particular serious incidents, but cannot investigate patterns of poor performance. The performance procedures have been introduced to fill this gap and have two main purposes: to protect the public and to give the deficient doctor the chance to improve.

The definition of "seriously deficient performance" is given by the GMC as:

a departure from good professional practice—whether or not it is covered by specific GMC guidance—sufficiently serious to call into question the doctor's registration.

133

The interpretation of this definition is also given as:

a doctor's registration may be called into question by repeated or persistent failure to comply with the standards appropriate to the work being done by the doctor, particularly where this places patients or members of the public in jeopardy. This may include repeated or persistent failure to comply with the GMC's guidance in good medical practice.

It is clear from these two statements that the GMC is only interested in doctors who are likely to place patients in serious jeopardy through their actual practice. The key principles of the procedures for assessment of performance have also been laid down by the GMC as:

- The assessment should be wide ranging, nor just focusing on the complaint.
- The process should be fair, open and transparent.
- The standard of assessment and adjudication should be consistent.
- The procedures should apply to all doctors in all types of practice.

Inevitably these procedures lead to new committees. Within the Fitness to Practise Division there is a committee called the Assessment Referral Committee, which will deal with queries from the screener, particularly if the doctor is reluctant to undergo assessment.

Following screening, the doctor is informed of the nature of any complaint that the GMC has received which is leading to the further assessment of general performance. It needs to be recognised that a pattern of poor performance needs to be established before the assessments are undertaken. The case is passed from the screener to a case coordinator, who is a doctor member of the GMC who chooses a panel of assessors. Recently the GMC has advertised publicly for people to apply to become assessors, and they are currently selecting these—both medical and lay. People chosen to become assessors have undergone a thorough training by the GMC on how to conduct the procedures. The case coordinator reports to another committee, called the Committee on Professional Performance, which is a new committee. This committee has the power to direct a doctor to undergo assessment, to access medical records, and to apply sanctions to a doctor's registration for non-cooperation, or as a result of an assessment. The committee determines formally whether the doctor's performance has been seriously deficient. If so, it imposes sanctions on the doctor's registration. This can either be as a condition on part of the practice, which can extend for 3 years, or it may be temporary suspension for 12 months, or in very difficult cases the suspension may be made indefinite.

The assessment panel usually will consist of two doctors from a similar specialty to the doctor under assessment, and a lay individual. The panel, having undertaken a formal assessment of the doctor in question, has to report back to the Committee on Professional Performance through the case coordinator. The GMC guidance is that the report given will have to address the following questions:

- In your opinion is the practitioner's performance satisfactory, so that no further action needs to be taken by the GMC in relation to the practitioner?
- In your opinion has the standard of the practitioner's professional performance been in any respect seriously deficient? If so, in what respects?
- In your opinion is the standard of the practitioner's professional performance likely to be improved by training?
- In your view should the practitioner:

  Be allowed to continue in unrestricted practice?
  Limit his/her practice in any way? If so, in what way?
  Cease all professional practice?

From these questions you will appreciate that at the end of the day the assessment leads to a peer review. The assessment will use a number of methods with variable validity and variable reliability. However, it should be remembered that the doctors whom we are concerned with here are those who will not fall onto a normal distribution curve of medical performance, but will be, as it were, off the left-hand end.

The lay assessor is a full member of the assessment panel and is there to represent the general public. The lay assessors have been chosen to bring in outside experience of assessment, and to provide public credibility to the process and its conclusions. One of the main methods of collecting evidence about a doctor's performance will be to conduct interviews with third parties, and it is expected that the lay assessor will lead these interviews.

135

The GMC has indicated that the assessment will consist of three stages. The first stage is to send to the doctor a portfolio to complete, which asks questions relating to his training and experience. The exact information required in the portfolio will vary from specialty to specialty, but within the portfolio there are open questions which allow the doctor to put forward any circumstances which may be affecting his performance. Many of the portfolios also include a self assessment of competence. The portfolios are designed to be non-judgmental, and are used to design a specific assessment for an individual. The attitude is that one can only judge the performance of a doctor on that doctor's particular practice. The assessment is not based on any college idealism. There are then two further stages of assessment:

- Phase 1 is designed to test performance and is to include a site visit to the doctor's actual practice.
- Phase 2 is designed to test competence and may, or may not, take place at the site of practice. It may involve objective testing, which is best conducted in appropriate centres.

On the whole it is expected that most doctors in the performance procedures will undergo phase 2 testing, but there is a mechanism whereby after the assessment in phase 1, the panel can report back to the Committee on Professional Performance and suggest that there is no case to answer and, therefore, the doctor does not have to undergo phase 2. However, for the sake of completing the assessment in a short period to relieve the doctor of the pressure that this attention will undoubtedly generate, it is expected that the arrangements for phase 2 testing will be agreed in advance of phase 1.

In phase 1 the following areas of practice are expected to be tested, but the exact method varies from specialty to specialty:

- Record keeping
- Case-based oral
- Practice organisation
- Observation of practice
- Audit of outcomes
- Third party interviews
- Structured interview with the doctor.

In phase 2 the following will be tested:

- Knowledge
- Clinical cases—assessor's material
- Clinical skills
- Consultation skills.

The third party interviews will be conducted by the lay assessor with the assistance of at least one of the doctors of the panel. These will be recorded by an independent stenographer, and it is expected that although they will fall short of a written formal statement by the interviewee, the interviewee will be asked to confirm the content. The people who will be interviewed will include persons related to the original complaints, remembering that a pattern of poor performance has to be established and, therefore, it is unlikely that individual patients will be involved, but other members of the public, such as from the Community Health Council, may well be interviewed. Other people to be interviewed will include people chosen by the doctor in question to a maximum (at present) of five people, and people chosen by the assessment panel. In general the specialty working parties who have been adapting the methodology to individual specialties have drawn up a list of suitable individuals for guidance. In radiology, for example, these would not only include radiological colleagues but also radiographers, nurses and clerical staff who work closely with the doctor. The aim is to obtain evidence from those people who actually work side by side with the doctor. The individual doctor may be accompanied by a "supporter" at all stages.

The GMC has set up working parties covering the specialties of practice, and all have been directed to produce written guidelines and formal formats to record the collection of evidence and to collate this in a report.

There have been many questions raised within the working parties regarding the legal basis of the procedures and of the protection that the GMC may be able to give to third party interviewees. Whatever the protection the GMC may provide to protect third parties from any legal action by the doctor regarding defamation of character, it cannot of course protect individuals from a worsening in relations due to the pressures that such procedures will bring, particularly where teamwork is normally expected.

It is recognised that no single test is infallible and the documentation is expected to demonstrate that evidence of bad practice has been collected and confirmed by a number of the methods outlined above.

The GMC recognises that in hospitals there are local procedures which should deal with the vast majority of such issues, and together with "clinical governance" the new procedure has forced a re-analysis of these in all trusts. The GMC is very keen not to become involved in contractual issues between a trust and its employees but is concerned to safeguard patients and to maintain standards through registration.

If a doctor is found to be seriously deficient through these procedures, it is the doctor's responsibility to arrange re-training, presumably with the help of college advisors and postgraduate deans. If this is not acceptable, then questions of early retirement or suspension from registration will come into play. Following a period of re-training, a doctor will undergo re-assessment with a further report to the Committee on Professional Performance.

4.8 The sick doctor

Contrary to their expectations doctors get sick. We have already seen that they are stressed and as a consequence have a high incidence of psychological illness, drug-related problems, alcohol abuse and suicide, quite apart from the normal gamut of physical illness. Ramirez found a 27% prevalence of psychiatric morbidity in consultants.[18] Their higher risk of suicide has been documented at 1.1–5.7 times that of the normal population.[19] They have a three times greater incidence of cirrhosis than the general population.[20]

Doctors with physical disease have a familiar and inappropriate set of responses to that disease.

- Denial.
- Failure to seek prompt advice.
- The use of advice gleaned from colleagues in the corridor.
- The avoidance of GPs and occupational health doctors.
- Self-diagnosis and self-medication.
- Unwillingness to take time off because of professional pressures and loyalty to colleagues. Doctors take only 1% of their time as sick leave compared with the NHS average of 5%,[21] and three-quarters of doctors admit to having worked when they felt so ill that their judgment was impaired.[22]

This is a very unhealthy situation. Nevertheless, consultants may use their experience and contacts to ameliorate the ill effects of this, but doctors in training do not have these options. Questionnaires and studies show unacceptable levels of physical and mental stress in doctors in training caused by the intensive workload and unfamiliar pressures of responsibility. Most of the calls received by the BMA Helpline are from doctors aged between 21 and 25.[23] There is little evidence that the "New Deal" has helped in this; it has merely increased the stress during the reduced working hours.

You may say that none of this is the medical manager's responsibility because there are supposed to be different channels for helping with these problems. The medical manager should, however, not ignore health issues in the staff who are her responsibility and that, of course, includes not only doctors but also nurses and others.

The medical manager must be involved because:

(1) She has a pastoral responsibility to the employees in her ambit, and

(2) Stress and illness, particularly psychological problems, drug and alcohol abuse, can impact on the effective care of patients, even their safety.

Her involvement may, however, be difficult as many employees, unfortunately, regard her as a Dickensian character usually trying to screw more work out of them and poised to fire them if they have problems. One way around this is to ensure that the specialty tutor or some other non-managerial clinician takes responsibility for the day-to-day welfare of trainees. Similarly for nurses and others there should be a specific named person with pastoral responsibility. The occupational health arrangements should be clearly advertised and counselling available. Most doctors prefer to be dealt with "off site" and should be aware of the BMA Stress Helpline (tel: 0645 200 169) and the National Counselling Service for Sick Doctors (tel: 0171 935 5982). This does not, of course, resolve the problem of doctors' unwillingness to admit to illness or to seek help. Cultural changes are necessary if this is ever to be resolved. Doctors must take more responsibility for their peers and have a preparedness to discuss illness perceived in colleagues. In addition, the system as a whole needs to pay particular attention to confidentiality where staff illness is concerned. This will require, for example, ensuring that test results are not generally available on the hospital computer system. All this, however, leaves a hiatus where patients are concerned. The clinical director or medical director is responsible for ensuring that sick doctors do not present a threat to patients. In this there is no difference from his responsibilities in relation to incompetent doctors. The current mechanisms to deal with the dangers sick doctors present are, however, somewhat confused. If sick doctors have insight and present themselves to the GP or the occupational health doctor, then it is that clinician's responsibility to advise the sick doctor that they are a risk to patients. If, however, doctors fail to present, refuse advice or have no insight into the problem, then one must rely on colleagues or other staff to sound the alarm. In that event the "three wise men" procedure comes into effect. "The three wise men" is the slang term for "a sub-committee of the Special Professional Panel set up under HC82/13". Although this is an old health circular it has not been cancelled and anyone involved in the difficulties surrounding the management of the sick doctor should read HC82/13 (I would not normally advise the reading of HCs as a pastime but this is an exception). In summary, the health circular says:

in paragraph 3

There should be a special professional panel set up by the medical executive committee consisting of members of the senior medical staff from which a small sub-committee should be appointed. The sub-committee should receive and take appropriate action on, any report of incapacity due to physical or mental disability including addiction. It does not have a duty to report back to the panel.

in paragraph 6

Information will normally be given in the first instance to one of the members of the panel but sometimes to the chairman of a clinical division. It may come from a variety of sources and may relate to medical or dental staff of any grade. It will usually be given by a colleague but may be from another discipline or from a general medical or dental practitioner.

in paragraph 8

The sub-committee should make such confidential enquiries as are necessary to verify the accuracy of any report. Whilst they are not required to establish positively that the possibility of harm to patients exists or to make a clinical diagnosis, nevertheless if they are satisfied the report has substance the practitioner should be told of its contents and be given the opportunity to be interviewed by the sub-committee ... If the sub-committee feel that the possibility of harm to patients cannot be excluded by the exercise of their influence ... they should bring the circumstances to the notice ... of the medical officer of the employing authority.

in paragraph 9

It is the responsibility of the officer of the employing authority who receives the report from the sub-committee under this procedure to decide what further investigations are necessary. If it appears that a question arises that the doctor's fitness to practice may be seriously impaired ... consideration should be given as to whether the circumstances might justify report to the registrar of The General Medical Council for consideration in accordance with the procedures of the council's health committee.

This remains one of the few formal responsibilities still vested in the medical committee of the hospital rather than the medical director. However, insofar as members of the panel might be held legally responsible for any harm to patients caused by a clinician who was unfit to practice and who had been notified to them yet the problem had been glossed over, it would seem to be prudent that the chairman of the panel should maintain close liaison with the medical director.

It ought not to be necessary to say so, but experience suggests that it is important to remember that the patient's welfare comes first, and that "buddy relationships" between clinicians which conceal incapacity are, in the long run, in nobody's interest.

One should not leave this subject without noting that most ill health in Health Service workers is psychological and much of that is a consequence of unsatisfactory working environment, overwork and poor organisation, all of which is in theory at least under the control of managers.

141

4.9 Professional and personal development

4.9.1 Professional development for clinicians generally

Professional development is a buzz term attracting much lip service though not always the commitment of a budget. As far as clinicians are concerned it is at its simplest Continuing Medical Education (CME), the refreshing of old skills and knowledge and the learning of new skills. It is an obligation inherent in the life of professionals, but if you see the annual returns detailing your colleague clinician's study leave you will probably be surprised at the range of uptake from the man who never misses a chance to fly away to meetings or slip off to his college (absences, which with other leave, not infrequently add up to more than 3 months of the year for academics) and contrast with the over-committed clinician who rarely misses a clinic and never takes study leave. The results from the 1996 CME review of the Royal Colleges of Surgeons of Edinburgh, England and Glasgow showed that 7% of surgeons who returned their forms did not achieve the necessary amount (25 hours) of study within their hospital and 13% failed to achieve enough external study time. As this was a self-reporting study it is probably an under-representation of inadequacy, as those who failed to reach the requirements were perhaps less likely to return their forms.[24]

The obligation to arrange CME remains a professional and ethical issue in Europe and the format of CME has changed little over the years. Yet we have no proof that hours spent in these traditional forms of CME, journal clubs, postgraduate meetings, deaths and complications meetings, professional group conferences, etc., actually improve our performance as clinicians. One study found that the number of reported CME hours correlated positively with *lower* competence!, an association of course, rather than a cause.[25] If then the medical manager is to put his hand to the oar to try and facilitate CME in his unit, he needs to remember that simply pressuring people into attending PGME meetings is not necessarily the correct answer. The cooperative and reflective medical team is itself an educational engine, but the crucial element is the efficiency of doctors' capacity for self-directed learning and that is not something which can be imposed. Actually, most doctors do not know what the phrase "self-directed learning" means or implies.

In spite of anxieties about the effectiveness of formal CME, its promulgation and measurement, though not of course its funding, continues to be a growth area in the Health Service. In the USA most of specialty board certification is now limited to 7–10 years, with re-certification necessary at the end of that time. This seemingly straightforward process has proved to be a financial and educational minefield and may not deliver any better results than other less formalised systems. As ever in spite of negative results from over the Atlantic the Department of Health is currently toying with the prospects for re-certification. Whatever the pundits might say about the value of enforced CME, it remains an obligation on medical managers to work to ensure that adequate time and funding is made available for such leave.

Educating clinicians about management

Professional development for clinicians in the form of "management training" is heavily proselytised. Trainees doubt that they will get a consultant post without having been on a "management course". This is sad, as a badly run course orientated towards business management seems often to raise antibodies to management in the very trainees who will be needed in the future to help manage the service. I have to express a bias here. I would personally prefer clearly to separate three types of management training:

(1) *NHS citizenship*, which is about how the NHS works.
(2) *Personal development*, which is about developing human skills which would be valuable in a management role but might currently be missing—communication, assertiveness, chairmanship, that sort of thing. This is covered later in this section.
(3) *Management training*, which deals with the specific skills needed to run the health business—personnel, finance, contracting, etc.

All doctors need (1), most will need some (2) and at some stage some may need (3), but certainly not at the undergraduate stage as has been proposed.[26]

The important part is the NHS citizenship training and that should indeed begin at undergraduate level and is often dressed up as a course in public health. This should improve the awareness of the mechanisms of the NHS, its financial and organisational constraints, ethical issues about rationing and a bit about practicalities such as equal opportunities. There is no reason why clinicians need go outside their own hospitals for this sort of training. It is probably more acceptable if it is merged with other educational activities within the hospital and it is the medical manager's obligation to arrange such sessions and coax clinicians to attend. A series of such sessions in our trust, aimed primarily at younger clinicians, has been gratifyingly well attended and better received than conventional wisdom would predict.

For the established clinician management training/professional development can usefully be tied to what he needs to know; that is to say a basic series of skills training should be made available (e.g. non-discriminatory interviewing, staff assessment, communication skills) and targeted education aimed at improving his comprehension of changes in the NHS (e.g. process improvement, audit, EBM, handling mergers).

4.9.2 Professional development for medical managers

Although it is fairly clear what professional development means for clinicians, it is uncertain exactly what it means in the context of the medical manager. One could say that it is simply something done by, to or for a medical manager to make her a better manager, but better at what?

For a medical manager such development can fall into one of two categories:

(a) Moulding the person to the corporate objectives
(b) Developing skills in the person to enable them better to fulfil their job as defined.

Moulding the person to fit the corporate plan

Most of the so-called management training proposals for doctors and students within the Health Service at present fall into this category. The idea is that if you show how the finances work, how the system works, what the constraints are and how to function in teams, if you explain to them the mechanics of purchasing and the inevitability of rationing then they will accept it and work better, more comfortably and quietly within the system. Whether that really is the outcome remains to be seen, but most hospital trainees now have some of this type of management training. Perhaps as a consequence some take a more understanding stance in relation to the running of the service but others do not and remain bitter recidivists. I doubt if it is known how many have been converted and, in view of the changing background against which such management development occurs, how can it be known? In the meantime, as an act of faith, we go on encouraging trainees and new consultants to go on management courses and perhaps, improperly, we provide the money for those courses with more readiness and enthusiasm than we do for their CME.

Developing the skills of the medical manager

It is worth asking whether there actually exists a body of knowledge and skill which a manager can learn and, indeed, does managerial competence exist as a measurable skill? It is an article of faith in the development business that such skills can be taught and learned, just as it is an article of faith that certain core competencies are needed to fulfil the job.

Core competencies

In their review of the management skills of clinical directors, Gatrell and White[27] listed the competencies (Table 4.3) and, commenting on their assessment of clinical directors in post based on 1400 questionnaire returns and 230 interviews, they noted that many clinical directors have met their own needs through experiencing problems and seeking answers and information themselves, but that "there are many who have learned to get by with a mixture of common sense, avoidance, information from peers and bluff". In addition to listing the skills required of a clinical director, they also listed those required for a medical director (Table 4.4). The difficult issue is how to decide which of the skills listed can and should be formally taught. Many are extensions of the skills already learned as a doctor. One needs to ask whether some of the competencies defined as desirable are really appropriate skills for a doctor-manager to learn, or whether their presence on the list is merely a reflection of an inappropriately defined job. Although in their report Gatrell and White indicate that the respondents to their questionnaires *asked* for training and development, I am not aware of any study that shows improved performance as a result of such formal management training. Lik Mui[28] looked at organisational problems experienced by medical directors and found that with time in post medical directors became better at the tasks, regardless of whether they had had training or not.

145

Table 4.3   Competencies required for a clinical director

- Implementing patient satisfaction indicators
- Negotiating contracts
- Monitoring business performance
- Business planning
- Managing a budget
- Generating income
- Handling official complaints
- Managing organisational crisis
- Using management information systems
- Problem solving and decision making
- Counselling colleagues and subordinates
- Chairing meetings
- Negotiating
- Conducting appraisal interviews
- Conducting selection interviews
- Delegating work to colleagues
- Acting as a figurehead
- Understanding and influencing organisational culture
- Managing professional reputation in the context of managerial work
- Implementing difficult non-clinical decisions
- Adopting an ethical management stance
- Handling uncertainty

(Reproduced from: Gatrell J, White T. *Medical Student to Medical Director—a development strategy*. NHS Training Division, 1995)

When he looked at personal problems (Table 4.5) he found less improvement with time.

One interpretation of the list of areas that medical directors found difficult is that their jobs as defined are too broad, their timetables too full. It is probably the job that should be altered in these circumstances, but if it is not then perhaps there is some

Table 4.4   Competencies required for a medical director

- Recruitment, selection of non-medical staff
- Pursuing equal opportunities
- Developing terms and conditions of employment
- Non-clinical staff training
- Staff appraisal
- Implementing decisions
- Disciplinary procedures
- Implementing patient satisfaction indicators
- Dealing with the media
- Negotiating
- Conducting interviews for grievance and discipline

(Reproduced from: Gatrell J, White T. *Medical Student to Medical Director—a development strategy*. NHS Training Division, 1995)

Table 4.5   Personal problems experienced by medical directors in relation to their posts

---

- Individual problems
- Reducing the difficulties for medical managers
- Lack of autonomy
- Dealing with difficult medical colleagues
- Gaining acceptability and trust of colleagues
- Managing the dual role of clinician and manager
- Time management
- Financial ability
- Lack of feedback on job performance
- Inadequate financial reward
- Impact on family
- Impact on career

(Reproduced from: Mui Lik D. MPhil Thesis, University of Oxford, 1997)

need for personal as distinct from professional development to help the manager cope.

Are the core competencies the right ones?
Current perceptions of development needs are probably wrong because they fix on skills and competencies needed to fulfil current jobs as described. Unfortunately, few organisations have asked if these job descriptions describe the jobs that clinicians really ought to be doing in management. The haphazard way in which clinical director and medical director posts were developed tended to lay too much stress on line management chores while neglecting the real value of medical managers to the process which is a bridge between medicine and the world of management. If that bridging role is the most important part of the medical manager's job, then we need to define the real core competencies to fulfil it. Chief among them is surely clinical credibility, and then the skills of leadership, persuasion, and manipulation; skills to do with acting as a first among equals, as an inspired messenger, and a wise arbiter. These are subtle skills perhaps not teachable, but they are certainly different from budget balancing, purchasing and personnel management skills, which occupy too much of clinical management time and training.

4.9.3 Personal development

Of course everyone needs to move on in life to evolve and mature. There is nothing new about that. Formalising the activity as

147

"personal development" has, however, become a management fad and I must confess to a heretical aversion to this for it has been an excuse for an almost wholly parasitic service industry to develop to support a fad. Personal development does not mean going to personal development courses; in general personal development, or the honing of generic skills, is a sophisticated process involving targeted education, re-energising through changing job patterns, visiting and sharing with colleagues and, lastly, "mentoring" within or outside one's own organisation. The personal developments needed are inherent in the list of generic skills which clinicians need but which are not formally taught.[29]

- Managing yourself (time management).
- Managing resources (usually money).
- Managing other people:
  being part of and leading a team
  managing meetings
  appointing and interviewing
  giving and taking feedback.
- Managing knowledge:
  lifelong learning (including the habit of self-directed learning)
  writing and publishing
  knowlege acquisition skills (libraries and computers)
  teaching skills.

In the Health Service we are not good at facilitating all these forms of personal development. Consultants in particular take on jobs like a country parson receiving a living and are expected to carry on a fixed pattern of work with the same momentum throughout life, ministering to the flock on the power of the spiritual lift-off that got them to the job in the first place. It is not enough but it does not mean we need a horde of quasi-professional advisers wanting us to pay them to be wiser than us about what is needed. That's triple jeopardy for the hospital. Pay the manager; pay the guru; pay for a locum. Targeted training for specific skills may be needed and there are outside consultancies who will organise these within NHS institutions. Professional organisations, the King's Fund and the royal colleges also arrange short and appropriate training courses.

Here is a selection of seminars featured at the Personal Development Show 1997 at Olympia in London:

- Down-shifting and Career Change.
- Personal Development—Your Competitive Edge.
- Revisioning Your Career.
- Explaining Neuro-Linguistic Programming.
- Dress for Success.
- Down-Shifting for Positive Life Balance.
- Why Do I Behave The Way I Do.
- Building Your Own Skills Passport.

In fairness I did not take a day off work and pay £10 at the door to benefit from all this, it might have been a wonderful life-enhancing experience but I doubt it. It will certainly have whipped up a lot of business for the business consultants, training providers, counsellors and "holistic" course providers who sponsored the meeting. Much of the personal development bonanza is a spin-off from the need for people to train "Me p.l.c." to survive in a world of short-term contracts and job mobility; where, as a Department for Education and Employment report recently found, one-third of employees have never been offered any job training. The NHS is different. We should manage personal development ourselves within the service and that should be available for all, not just managers. Interviews and questionnaires show that what attracts many people to jobs or makes them leave is the opportunity for further education. A *professional* (as distinct from personal) development within the job ought to be provided routinely by the trust. Beyond that the sort of mutual support networks and mentoring arrangements that primitive cultures enjoy as a routine should be explicitly set up or at least supported. This is particularly important for medical managers who may feel isolated from their natural peer group and not fully accepted or even supported by the other managers.

References

1 Weightman J. Working in teams. In: *Managing People in the Health Service*. London: Institute of Personnel and Development, 1996, pp. 36–50.
2 Belbin R. *Management Teams*. Oxford: Butterworth, 1981.
3 NAHAT. *Hospital and Community Health Services Medical Recruitment Survey*.
4 Clay B. Flexible training. *BMJ Classified* 23 May:2–3.
5 The Audit Commission. *The Doctor's Tale*. London: HMSO, 1995.

6 White A, Gattrell J. Appointing SpRs and getting it right first time. *Clin Management* 1997;**6**:9–14.

7 Donaldson L. Conflict, power and negotiation. In: Simpson J, Smith R, eds. *Management for Doctors*. London: BMJ Books, 1995.

8 Courtis J. *Bluff Your Way in Management*. Horsham: Ravette Publishing, 1992, p. 40.

9 Weightman J. *Managing People in the Health Service*. London: Institute of Personnel and Development, 1996, p. 114.

10 Eisenberger R, Cameron J. Detrimental effects of rewards. Reality or myth. *Am Psychol* 1996;**51**:1153–66.

11 Armstrong M. *Managing Rewards Systems*. Milton Keynes, Buckinghamshire: Open University Press, 1993, pp. 75–97.

12 Bloor K, Maynard. Rewarding health care teams. *Br Med J* 1998;**316**: 569.

13 Berne E. *Games People Play*. London: Andre Deutsch, 1966.

14 Association of Trust Medical Directors. *When Things Go Wrong*. British Association of Medical Managers, 1997.

15 Macgregor D. *The Human Side of Enterprise*. New York: McGraw-Hill, 1960. Cited by Weightman J. *Managing People in the Health Service*. London: Institute of Personnel and Development, 1996, p. 120.

16 McKevitt C, Morgan M. Illness doesn't belong to us. *J R Soc Med* 1997;**90**:491–5.

17 Annotation. *Br Med J* 1995;**311**:1594.

18 Ramirez AJ *et al*. Mental health of hospital consultants, the effects of stress and satisfaction at work. *Lancet* 1996;**347**:724–8.

19 Lindeman S *et al*. A systematic review on gender-specific suicide mortality in medical doctors. *Br J Psychol* 1996;**168**:274–9.

20 Brandon S. *Sick Doctors: a conspiracy of friendliness*. Keele: Mercia, 1995, pp. 18–24.

21 Seccombe L, Patch A. *Health at Work in the NHS: key indicators*. Final Report. Brighton: Institute of Employment Studies, University of Sussex, 1994.

22 Waldron HA. Sickness in the medical profession. *Ann Occup Hyg* 1996;**40**:391–6.

23 Richards T. Disillusioned doctors. *Br Med J* 1997;**314**:1705–6.

24 Results of 1996 CME Scheme. *Ann R Coll Surg Engl* 1998;**80**(Suppl): 9.

25 Caulford PG *et al*. Physician incompetence: specific problems and predictors. *Acad Med* 1993;**270**(Suppl):16–18. Cited by Holm HA. Quality issues in CME. *Br Med J* 1998;**316**:621–4.

26 Hornick P *et al*. Should business management training be part of medical education? *Ann R Coll Surg Engl* 1997;**79**(Suppl):200–1.

27 Gatrell J, White T. *Medical Student to Medical Director—a development strategy*. NHS Training Division, 1995.

28 Mui Lik D. MPhil Thesis, University of Oxford, 1997.

29 Pencheon D. Development of generic skills. *Br Med J* 1998;**316**(Suppl 12):2–3.

5 How the NHS Works

Thus God knows the world because he conceived it in his mind, as if from the outside, before it was created and we do not know its rules, because we live inside it, having found it already made.

(Umberto Eco[1])

5.1 Politics, planning and doctors

The NHS as we are often reminded is one of the world's largest businesses; as big as the Red Army they used to say. For those of us inside it is a challenging task trying to see how it works, for it works not just as a structured hierarchical command system like the Red Army but as a subtle, self-motivating, self-adjusting mechanism. Delivering healthcare to the nation was always so both before and after Aneurin Bevan re-badged it as The National Health Service. The wonder of the NHS is the way in which this adaptation and adjustment occurs. Politicians who have tried to change the NHS radically against the flow of this organic re-adjustment have found the organism not very biddable. The determinism that rules the NHS is truly organic. By that I mean that there are extensive homeostatic mechanisms quietly at work, repair processes that work effectively without central instruction, even as the parts age, decay or are damaged the whole survives. Indeed, if the totality of central management nationally and locally were to disappear tomorrow the system would remain in responsive, level flight for months or even years; some say it would soar!

5.1.1 The grand axis

By the grand axis of the NHS I mean the defined bureaucratic common structure that transfixes the system from top to bottom which like the "grand axe" of monumentalist French planners is intended to give a rationalist coherence to the whole.

The neat hierarchical "organogram" of the NHS starts at the top with the Secretary for Health as agent of cabinet government and then cascades relentlessly down through the ministers, the NHS Executive, regional outposts, the boards of trusts and through their executive committees to clinical directors and thus to the hapless workers in the service pinned to their desks you might think by the weight of this superstructure. But, of course, it does not work like that—the workers are not hapless, the patients are not passive. True there is a main core of command and control but it is modulated by other forces. That modulation of negative and positive feedback that affects the seemingly simple structure is what creates the stability of the system. More of that later. For the moment we need to consider the basic policy-making forces at work on the central core and the position of doctors in the system.

5.1.2 Formulation of health policy

The formulation of health policy and its execution within a NHS makes a wondrous playground for social scientists and political theorists and for those constructing dead-end courses in minor universities. The complexity and subtlety of the subject confounds accurate or constructive analysis so the field is wide open for historians and theorists; but does all this matter to the working doctor and the new medical manager? Not really, except that she needs to understand that the health policy whose end points will embroil her in a lot of sweat, toil and tears is not the product of a tidy intellectual process where sound facts are processed through a system built to satisfy a clear set of ideological and practical principles. In reality the facts are fragile as any clinician who has matched the official data to the real will know, and the ideological principles are broad brush: "to supply a comprehensive Health Service open to all free at the point of delivery" (and you might add "and at as little cost as possible to the taxpayer"). Beyond these simple principles and a few short-term political fashions such as "market forces", health policies and priorities are a set of compromises between the Department of Health, the Treasury, party ideologues, the BMA, the universities, the royal colleges, the patients even. A "complex web of mutual dependencies supporting a shifting assembly of pacts and bargains, both formally negotiated and tacitly understood,"[2] or to quote another writer "policy paradigms are a curious mix of psychological assumptions, scientific concepts, value commitments, social aspirations, personal beliefs and administrative constraints".[3] However capricious policy may eventually seem to the end user, it must in addition be formulated within inescapable and constantly fluctuating constraints such as demographic change increasing the number of the elderly, European law changing workers' hours, changing economic growth, the arrival of AIDS and immigrants, new technology, fashions in consumer demand and so on, some quite unexpected and inexplicable, like the recent inexorable rise in acute hospital admissions. When one tries to make sense of the policy-making which takes account of all these processes working together, a few threads can be identified which are reasonably consistent, forming what Harrison describes as "the shared version of health policy analysis". The major anatomical features of that shared version as summarised and carefully referenced by Harrison[4] are:

- Healthcare politics are incrementalist, i.e. slow or of narrow scope rather than systematic or radical.
- The policy process is usually one of "partisan mutual adjustment" (PMA) in which no one player can impose change alone and several can veto it.
- Within the PMA process the medical profession wields enormous influence.
- The position of lay health authority and trust board members is weak.
- The position of consumer organisations is even weaker.
- The "Centre" (i.e. the Department of Health/NHS Executive) has little direct control over the implementation of most national policies.
- The role of senior managers is usually reactive with the emphasis on "fire fighting", diplomacy, conflict avoidance, and consensus seeking.
- Policy inertia is exacerbated by the complexity of the Health Service as a whole.
- The whole complex and slow-moving edifice has been underpinned by an extremely durable political consensus, internally between the government and medical profession and externally between the government and the people about the primacy of a NHS as an institution.

Whether this cassoulet of diverse ingredients makes for a satisfying and warming dish or an unsatisfactory mush suitable for

153

no one's palate is a matter of taste and expectation, but its various ingredients are crucial to the homeostatic controls that work on the Health Service.

Mrs Thatcher certainly did not like the taste, so in the infamous "Working for Patients"[5] she added piquancy in the shape of market forces, competition, the purchaser/provider split and fundholding GPs. Her interventions were often unwelcome not only because of their dogmatism and lack of consensuality, but also because they disturbed the equilibrium of the system. In addition crucially they failed to address the issue of the proper funding of the service, the very pressure that had stimulated the changes. Many of the changes trumpeted in "Working for Patients" were counter-productive to the economic and practical needs of the service, and within a short time of their promulgation, and while medical and non-medical managers were struggling to implement the changes, commentators were already drafting the obituaries. "The NHS . . . might be seen as the unfortunate victim of a mugging that ought never to have occurred. Saddled at great cost with a market apparatus that nobody really wanted . . . it faces a bleak future."[6] Early analyses of the effects of "competition" in the NHS show no evidence of improved cost effectiveness. This is so even if the direct costs of the internal market are excluded from the equation. Transaction costs in the NHS were about 5% in the 1980s and rose to 12% with the arrival of the internal market.[7,8]

By contrast, individualised and marketised welfare has a habit of introducing more choice for the few at the expense of lower quality service for the many.[9]

Even those who have an enthusiasm to denigrate or dismantle the effects of "Working for Patients" ought to be aware of the radical changes it seeded into the soil of the NHS culture:

- The concept and the reality that change was possible in the Health Service.
- Change can be implemented quite quickly.
- It is feasible and probably preferable to separate the businesses of defining health care needs (note that I do not say "purchasing") from the business of providing the care.
- The debate about priorities has become easier.
- The measurement of cost and quality have become everyday concerns at all levels in the service.

154

In spite of that "Working for Patients" is slowly working its way out of agenda papers and into the history books to become just another tuck in the fabric of the Service.

The features of NHS policy making which make for stability also make it difficult to influence, for there is no prince to flatter, no dictator to buy, no chieftain's pow-wow to attend, no obvious way to change things, such that there seems to be an inevitability about most Health Service policy when it reaches the working clinical manager which tends to imply inalterability. However this should not deter the clinical manager from speaking out, because coherent comment and complaint really does alter the detail when implementing health policy and may contribute to a political environment which eventually allows change. Some of the most dysfunctional effects of the "Working for Patients" reforms were quickly undone by the incoming Blair government in 1997, not just for ideological reasons but because they had heard the congruent criticisms that had come up from the lower tiers of managers and users.

Figure 5.1 shows some examples of the forces at work on the grand axis of central command and which can modulate health policy. While I have described above the influences as being essentially constructive, there are times when the sheer number of influences working within an organisation as complex as the NHS can frustrate the achievement of *any* end point at all, let alone the right one. An example of this is shown in Figure 5.2, which is the chart Dr Susan Atkinson (Director of Public Health, South Thames Region) constructed to try to understand the forces at work in medical manpower planning following the establishment of Local Medical Workforce Advisory Groups (LMWAGs) in 1996.

In the midst of all this it is worth looking more closely at the relationship between the government/Department of Health and the medical profession, because it is that relationship which has thrown up the principle that clinicians in management are "a good thing".

Relationships between government and doctors

As I conceive it the function of the Ministry of Health is to provide the medical profession with the best and most modern apparatus of medicine, and to enable them freely to use it, in accordance with their training, for the benefit of the people of

155

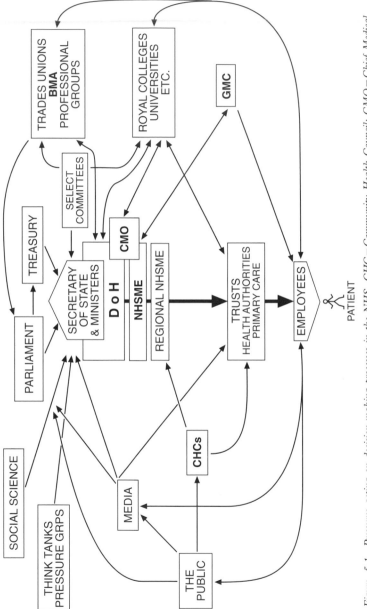

Figure. 5.1 Pressures acting on decision-making processes in the NHS. CHC=Community Health Council; CMO=Chief Medical Officer; DoH=Department of Health; GMC=General Medical Council; NHSME=NHS Management Executive.

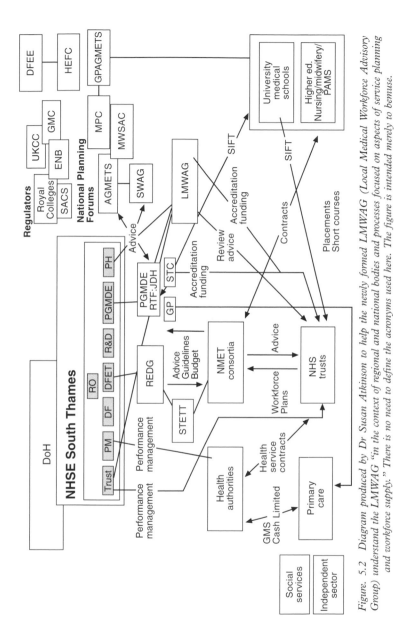

Figure. 5.2 Diagram produced by Dr Susan Atkinson to help the newly formed LMWAG (Local Medical Workforce Advisory Group) understand the LMWAG "in the context of regional and national bodies and processes focused on aspects of service planning and workforce supply." There is no need to define the acronyms used here. The figure is intended merely to bemuse.

this country. Every doctor must be free to use that apparatus without interference from secular organisations.

(ERNEST BEVIN in the House of Commons 30/4/46
Hansard Col. 52)

Ever since the deals that Aneurin Bevan did with the doctors at the inception of the NHS in 1946, there has been an unspoken pact between the profession and a sequence of governments and the Department of Health. The culture of the pact was that the Government/Department of Health would act centrally to set the political agenda and define the funding available, but would leave the peripheral side of the business to the doctors who would decide how best to deliver care, how to respond to changes in medical advances, and even deal with politically sensitive issues such as rationing. In the last 10 years that pact has taken a beating and it is worth questioning whether it still exists.

The more political or less kind social scientists have interpreted the profession's stance in this compact with the government as being essentially self-protective, defensive, conservative and cynical—frustrating all moves that might diminish the profession's power, influence or income. Doctors themselves by contrast see their public role as being the sole protector for the patient against a succession of governments bent only on reducing costs. The doctor as "mother tiger". Both these views can, of course, be true! What is certain is that there has always been a degree of what social scientists call "liberal corporatism"[10] Liberal corporatism describes a process in which to ease the business of running complex organisations the government abrogates responsibilities for some of its tasks to certain moderate and well-organised groupings who it can expect to control their members and liaise constructively with the public. The medical profession is one such.

Until the late 1970s the marriage was acceptably harmonious, free of too many arguments about money, even though as early as 1953 a committee had been set up to to try to control expenditure on the NHS. Money has since then been the root of all difficulties. First dramatically in the late 1970s when doctors questioned the government's stewardship of the budget not only in relation to their own salaries but also in terms of the allocation for health care itself. This was eventually brought to the brink of "industrial action". While the salaries issue was, to some extent, resolved the general funding of the Health Service has never been resolved.

The principles of cash limits and resource allocation did not resolve the problem nor did the importation of managerialism as a consequence of the Griffiths Report of 1983.[11] To control costs the government and the Department of Health had to make inroads into areas which the traditional compact had left to doctors. Managers and markets do not alone control costs and where costs continually outrun the supply of money doctors (who are usually the first and the loudest in complaint) are perceived as the agents of overspending. In taking over areas previously left to doctors the attack has been on two fronts, both of which are based on the principle that it is doctors who commit resources and spend money.

(1) The basis on which they do this must be questioned—hence evidence-based medicine and managed care (see Section 6.7).
(2) Doctors must be "on board" so that they understand the finite nature of available funds and take direct managerial responsibility for the use of those funds—hence the clinical director.

Therefore with the arrival of the clinical director and the fund-holding GP we have a new and formal extension of the longstanding pact of liberal corporatism, where it is understood that an elite of doctors can be recruited to deliver budget targets and bring pressure to bear in controlling costs in areas such as length of stay, use of drugs, application of new technology, etc. Whether the invention of clinical management can deliver the Holy Grail of an affordable Health Service remains to be seen, but it seems unlikely. The history of the NHS is one of frantic and every-varying attempts at maximal cost containment with minimal political damage, while holding on to the basic tenets that underpin the service. Whether the time is yet ripe for a government to address the basic problem of underfunding rather than merely plan another "reform" also remains to be seen.

The obsession with control

The combined effect of the near total dependence of Health Service Funding on central taxes distributed through the Treasury which ensures a continuing and desperate search for financial stability, together with the belief that the front-line professionals are the agents of wilful and inappropriate spending coupled with a loss of respect for the autonomy of professional groups, has trapped recent

159

governments into an ever-tightening demand for control while publicly sounding off about devolvement of power. This is politely described as the move from "public administration" to "public management". As with traditional administration, public management is often offered as a set of neutral reforms for increasing the efficiency and responsiveness of public service delivery in a more complex economic and social environment. However, as several writers have argued, this perspective should be regarded with suspicion, not least because public management carries with it its own set of values and assumptions which if cultural change is to be achieved may be used to supplant those of the administrative cultures it seeks to replace or control.[12] Simon Jenkins in his book "Accountable to None"[13] has documented in detail the development of this trend during the years of Thatcherite government driven by a relentless desire for cost savings. In that quest any financial risk was to be minimised and the delegation to the periphery and to professionals by which the service had previously been managed became suspect. As Jenkins remarks:

> The act of delegation requires the delegator to take risks, especially in the short term. Yet politics is about minimizing risk, avoiding bad publicity, watching out for banana skins. By centralizing decision, a minister can give himself the illusion that he is minimizing risk. He may be but he is blanketing decision in a fog of caution and irresolution.

The desire to control—the old Stalinist reflex of governments of all colours—is not reflected in good management practice in the world outside which stresses the importance of empowering the functional units within an organisation, giving them leeway in achieving or even exceeding the corporate objectives. As a medical manager you will see repeated examples of the caution and slowness that characterises the processes within the Health Service bent primarily on control. For example, the empty but staffed operating theatre made so by a system that demands pre-authorisation of extra-contractual referrals or will not "allow" elective surgery to be admitted beyond a contracted number.

The consequence of a demand for control is a crippling bureaucracy, the issuing of directives without proper consultation and the endless demand for "returns", reams of neurotically collected data attempting to ensure that directives are being observed: "is audit being done?", "how heavy was each breast biopsy?", "how long was it from the diagnosis to the implementation of thrombolysis?", etc. etc., and more recently: "how many managers do you have?", "how much do they cost?", "how are you going to reduce their numbers?" This last is indeed the ultimate irony in that the mouth is wishing to bite the hand it commissioned to feed it! Meanwhile as Jenkins ruefully concludes in his chapter on the Health Service:

> . . . the centralization of the service left an uneasy feeling that a professional relationship of trust between patient and doctor and hospital and community had been broken. A new and cruder accountability had been put in place, to a vague concept of national efficiency and to a nervous minister to parliament.

Since that was written a new streak is detectable in the arguments (especially since the Bristol paediatric cardiac surgery fiasco), namely that the medical profession needs to be controlled managerially not just because doctors are incapable of financial discipline but also because they are clinically inefficient, heedless of quality, and deaf to consumers' needs. The compact such as it is between government and professions hardly exists in this scenario and the clinical director becomes merely "pig in the middle" between controller and the controlled.

The clinical director as "pig in the middle"

Historians may, in due course, record the failure of clinical management. If they do so it may be because we have tried to load the clinical manager with two further objectives in addition to the control of expenditure. The other targets being delivery of quantity and quality. Unfortunately these three requirements are frequently irreconcilable, and in attempting to reconcile the delivery of quality and quantity at decreased cost the volunteer clinical director may come close to extinction as a breed and the compact between the government and the profession will need to be re-worked yet again.

There are no doubt those who say that the power of doctors should and can be so curtailed by management such that no further compact is necessary. The power of doctors has in essence always been the possession of the magic of medicine. Only they can say the spells and only they occupy what has been called "the secret garden". The automation of clinical management by EBM-driven protocols and the steady denigration of professionalism by those outside has not yet, as Klein claims, shrunk the secret garden to

161

the size of a window box.[14] In spite of the rise in complaints and litigation, surveys show that patients still believe the doctors are more likely to look after their interests than are managers, politicians or purchasers; so long as that perception remains the magician will need to be given a place.

The current or a future government may wish to let the financial imperatives force the pace and not bother to make accommodations with the profession; but this seems unlikely. At the very least they will need to take into account the view of medical managers, particularly if those managers can show themselves to be cognisant and sympathetic to the realities of funding and organising a comprehensive Health Service. If then the medical manager remains an entity in the NHS he or she is likely to define and lead the professional end of any continued compact.

One should not leave this arena on too sour a note. The management of the NHS has been bedevilled by its very complexity, its size, the lack of adequate data about how it's working and what it needs to do, confounded by unremitting and ungovernable change. It is reasonable to suppose that even had it been played by different people to different rules the results would have been much the same or worse.

5.2 NHS finance

What a tragedy it is to live in an age of such consummate cost consciousness.

(B. BRYSON[15])

As medical manager you will spend too much time explaining to staff that although you deprecate the shortage of money in the NHS and understand their desires for more, there is nothing you yourself can do to increase that sum of money, and they will need to grapple with the reality of a finite budget. It is not an argument you will enjoy promulgating but you will do it so often that it is helpful to know enough of NHS finances to understand why things are as they are.

5.2.1 Where the money comes from

The money which funds the NHS comes predominantly from general taxation with a much lesser contribution from the National

Insurance Scheme, a fraction from prescription charges and small amounts from private practice within NHS institutions and miscellaneous sources such as the sale of land. The majority thus comes directly from the Exchequer. The sums involved are huge (£44 billion in 1997) and represent about 14% of public spending which itself represents 43% of the gross domestic product (the GDP = what we earn as a nation + what as a nation we borrow [the PSBR (public sector borrowing requirement)]). Forty years ago NHS expenditure as a percentage of GDP was a mere 3%, but it rose rapidly in the 1970s and since then has remained remarkably stable at between 5% and 6%. Nevertheless in times of difficulty all of us within the NHS like to point out that the NHS claims a smaller percentage of GDP than almost all our Western European colleagues and about half of what is claimed in the USA. Put another way, in 1994 the UK spent £789 per head on healthcare, Germany £1552, and the USA £2285[16] (Figure 5.3). A public health guru or savvy Treasury official might respond that the quality or even the quantity of care that the money buys in the UK is, in fact, comparable to that in equivalent countries,

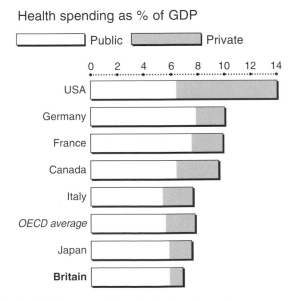

Figure 5.3   Total health care spending of a selection of countries as a percentage of GDP (Gross Domestic Product). The figures include both public and private expenditure. (Data source: OECD, 1995.)

163

and that many health indices such as access to basic care, life expectancy and perinatal mortality are better in the UK than in comparable countries (Figure 5.4). But at what cost? An overworked workforce frequently demoralised by the insufficiency of finance *vis-à-vis* a decent environment for them and their patients; a slow, inadequate response to advances in healthcare; real and continuing deficiencies in psychiatric and community care and extensive covert rationing.

From their insulated fastnesses the public health theoretician and the Treasury official may continue to conclude that funding is adequate, but the perception from the front-line is that it is not. Although national surveys show the majority of UK citizens are generally very content with "their" Health Service, international comparators however show that there is a relationship between the spending per head on healthcare and the users' satisfaction (Figure 5.5).

5.2.2 How the money is allocated

There are two sides to Health Service finance: the allocation of money, "the *supply* side", and the demands for its use, "the *demand* side."

In defining the supply side the government is subject to the general political pressures on it. Education and health are currently in fashion, defence is not. Social security is not in fashion, quite the opposite, but it is largely uncontrollable and is the greatest demand on the public purse. The annual exercise in settling the total amount available to the NHS in theory takes account of medical advances, the funding implications of government policies as well as inflation, but the allocations for these are rarely what the real figures would demand (Figure 5.6), and there is a further reducing effect in that a percentage is also removed for anticipated "productivity gains". This productivity gain is expected to be made every year, which leaves the Treasury with a happy prospect that some time during the next century the cost of providing healthcare will approach zero!

Once the overall sum for the year is allocated to the NHS it is deemed to be fixed. In the jargon the service is "cash limited". However, within the service itself not all budgets are cash limited. Hospital services are but GP prescribing is currently not. Once the total is agreed centrally the central costs of running the NHS are

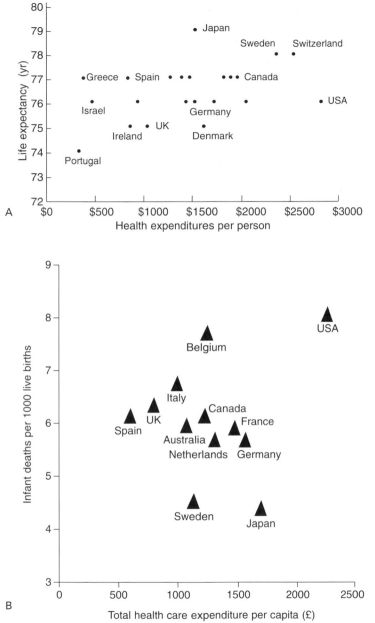

Figure 5.4 (A) National health expenditures per capita in relation to life expectancy. (Data source: World Bank Development Report, 1993) (B) National health expenditure per capita in relation to infant mortality. (Data cited in: Br Med J 1997;315:568)

165

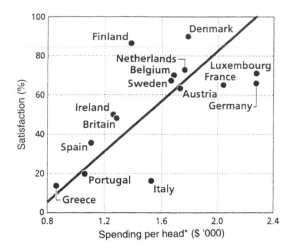

*Figure 5.5   Health spending and public satisfaction with health services. *AV purchasing power parity.*

deducted and the remainder distributed to health authorities, although some is "top sliced" for special areas such as HIV and other pet projects. The mechanics of allocation to regions and within regions to specific districts and trusts is determined by complex formulae, the validity and application of which are hotly argued by those who see themselves as doing badly as a result of

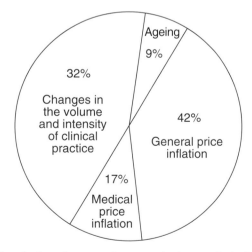

Figure 5.6   Contribution of separate factors to the increase in healthcare spending. (Data source: Muir Gray, Evidence-Based Healthcare. Figure 2.5)

the allocations; which is pretty much everybody. The mechanics of allocation change regularly in an attempt to make it simpler or more equitable. Since 1990 the process has been one of resident/ capitation-based funding. Each region's population is "weighted" to reflect the age profile within the region and the demands that its population place on the Health Service. These "capitation rates" are based on the estimated expenditure per head for different age groups. The age-weighted populations are adjusted by the SMR (standardised mortality ratio) and certain geographical supplements are then added, such as "London weighting" to reflect the higher costs for staff living in the capital. Social deprivation factors are being considered but are not currently built into the formula. The derivation of the formulation and its application is modified to some extent by political considerations and the difficulty of taking money from one part of the country to give to another. Academics who deal in these matters are never satisfied and Sheldon has pointed out that, in fact, the use of a much simpler formula based simply on population size, age and SMR would be just as good.[17] The rules governing allocation are reasonably fixed but the latitude in them allows for separate districts to feel hard done to. Poor and deprived areas seem always to lose out. The position of teaching trusts is also disputed. Those outside, of course, consider them over resourced. There is, at present, a detailed dissection of teaching hospital costs underway to separate the costs of teaching and of research from those of service to make them more explicit and thus more accountable. Unfortunately, as anyone in a teaching hospital knows, the three faces of teaching hospital medicine are so intricately interwoven that no accurate division is achievable, and any dissection is likely to show the whole body to be starved rather than obese.

Allocations are rendered even more opaque by the top slicing of money for specific areas such as educational budgets from which trainees are partly paid. After all this the money is then, of course, not allocated directly to the provider units but to the purchasers who go round another complex set of exercises as part of the contracting process which decides who will do what and who gets the money. In this, the third turn of the merry-go-round, cost and quality of service are taken into account and purchasing is also used as a vehicle to force changes in the configuration of providers, to encourage mergers, etc. The process is summarised in Figure 5.7.

PURCHASER   PROVIDER

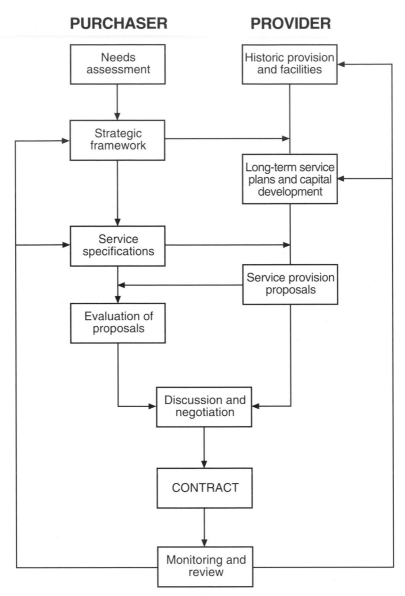

Figure 5.7   Cross-relationships between the purchaser and provider in the contracting process.

Into this muddy whirlpool we must also throw the effects of fundholding by GPs and the often quirky way that they in turn purchase care. GP fundholders, the *bêtes noires* of the Labour Party in opposition but now being redressed in the new respectable costume of primary care groups, are set to become another agent in the cost control and budget allocation chain.

The trail from tax-payers' pockets via the Treasury, Department of Health, NHS Executive and purchasers to the hospitals that care for them is more convoluted than the ways a drug baron uses to launder his proceeds. There is thus no way that any medical manager would be able to justify to her staff whether the budget they are working to represents a fair allocation or not. There must be simpler ways, but the simplest and most transparent, such as the "fee for item of service" which is much put about by disenchanted staff, is unacceptable because that mechanism takes away the ability to manipulate and to cash limit the service.

One should not deny the importance of getting allocation right both at a macro and a micro level. Thomas Getzen, a US Health Economist, says that in health economics "Allocation, Allocation, Allocation" is what is important, echoing the estate agent who when asked what are the three most important factors in determining property value replies "Location, Location, Location".[18] If the *right patient*, is going to get the *right treatment* in the *right place* at the *right time*, allocation needs to be accurate, adequate and forceful. The NHS tends to fall down on all three.

5.2.3 Why can't more money be raised?

So long as the government of the day believes the efficiency and productivity of the NHS is substandard and could be improved, while it believes it can weather the little squalls about health that constantly blow through the media there is no incentive radically to review the funding basis of the NHS. Each new government is encouraged to review that funding but never does. If it were to, what options would it have?

- A rise in general taxation levels.
- A hypothecated tax, i.e. one earmarked for health.
- A reallocation of spending from other ministries to health.
- Increased and new charges for services, e.g. £10 for visiting a GP, £25 a day for time in hospital.

- Withdrawal of funding from healthcare retreating to a safety net for the poor or to an emergencies only service.
- Part payment leaving enforced personal insurance to pick up the remainder of the cost.

None of these, of course, commends itself and the option of the 1990s, money from the National Lottery, makes but a tiny dimple in the problem. Interestingly the public is not as averse to changes in the funding of the NHS as you would think, it is the insiders who are more likely to revere the founding Marxist principle of a free service. A Mori poll in 1998 commissioned by Age Concern showed that three-quarters of those polled still believed in a free Health Service but 39% thought that those who failed to follow medical advice should not receive free treatment and 44% thought non-essential items should be covered by insurance rather than the NHS. No government has yet shown any sign of withdrawal from the full commitment to the NHS and the spectre of raising taxes has no appeal to a government with any sense of electoral survival. Each government therefore falls back on the only real option remaining to it, cost containment, reassured by the know-ledge that almost any extra funding that was identified would anyway be quickly swallowed in line with Parkinson's Second Law that "expenditure rises to meet income" and the complaints of underfunding would only be deferred because demand seems to be inexorable (Figure 5.8).

5.2.4 Demand

The government sees the outputs of the healthcare process continually rising, more people are treated year on year, but these outputs fall short of *demand* which is almost certainly short of *need*. The need for healthcare far from diminishing as Bevan hoped in 1947 has grown. NHS activity has risen from 7 million finished consultant episodes (FCEs) in 1990 to 10.6 million in 1996/97. All this of course probably represents not a sicker population but simply changed expectations of health.

The use of emergency FCEs rose by 4.4% in 1996/97 over 1995/96 and the number of outpatient attenders increased from 10.8 million in 1995/96 to 11.2 million in 1996/97. The General Household Survey of 1996/97, when compared to that of 1972,

170

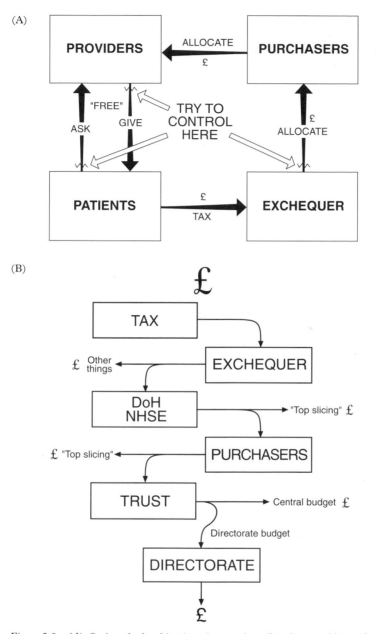

Figure 5.8 (A) Options for breaking into the taxation–allocation–provision cycle. (B) Laundering the tax-payers' money. No one working in a clinical directorate can judge the fairness of allocation because of the complexity of the process.

showed a doubling in the percentage of the population who categorise themselves as suffering from an acute illness.

Behind all this lurks The Waiting List so beloved by the media as an indicator and still standing at well over 1 million. It will always be impossible to match financial inputs to health outputs for a variety of reasons. For example:

- New technology usually yields less health gain per pound spent than does old technology (Figure 5.9).
- In spite of all the effort by government and hospitals, the real productivity of cases treated per pound spent has gone down.
- Calman, New Deal, new technology, The Patient's Charter, time spent in bureaucratic activities, increased contact time with patients, audit are all lowering real productivity.

Quite simply there are more staff and yet we see less patients each per year and we spend more money on each one of them.[19]

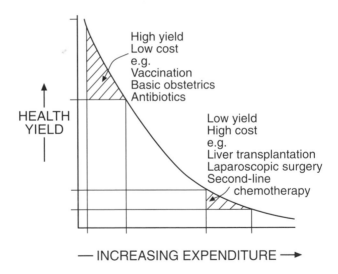

Figure 5.9   Higher levels of expenditure on health services do not normally produce as much health gain per £ as do lower levels.

5.2.5 Hidden unmet costs

A worrying feature of the NHS that the budget-holding manager will quickly discover is an invisible line in the budget. It should be there and should include the costs thus far unmet of "backlog maintenance" plus the cost of obviating clinical and other risks already known about and the cost of replacing equipment that is obsolete but for which there is no replacement plan. There are other things to add here but these are the big three. No figure exists for the national total in this invisible line. An NHS Confederation Survey released in 1998 concluded that at least £3 billion was needed just for essential maintenance.

5.2.6 Revenue, capital and capital charges

Revenue is the day-to-day housekeeping money that is spent on patient care. *Capital* is the separately allocated sum used for large items of expenditure; strictly defined as anything capable of being used for more than a year and costing more than £5000, so all buildings and most equipment are *capital*. The capital budget is allocated to trusts and districts and some is retained centrally. The mechanics of allocation and expenditure also have to take into account depreciation and are just as complex as the processes for allocating revenue. Trusts are required to pay back a notional interest on capital to ensure efficiency in its use so that, for example, we do not hang on to empty buildings or have more pieces of equipment than are needed. It is, in short, to ensure that we "sweat our assets". It was also perceived by many as a Conservative government's first steps towards "privatisation" of the Health Service. In the NHS capital cannot in theory be used as revenue and vice versa.

The issue of the financing of the Health Service will remain, as it always has been, an unedifying and untidy spectacle. The government desperate to limit costs will avoid talking about inputs and talk about outputs. Government spokesmen will always talk about how many more of this or that have been dealt with in the last year without observing whether that met need. Providers will only fix on the outputs they might provide if finance were sufficient and purchasers will try to get all the outputs they think they need for the input that has been allocated. Battles will be fought largely in the media. It is as Klein has observed a "dialogue of the deaf". In the same essay Klein goes on to point out that any narrative on the Health Service will always "revert to the built in tensions that spring directly from the original failure to base the funding of the

173

NHS on anything more solid than the shifting sands of political fashions and governmental preferences". A failure which would, he predicts, allow him "to describe a climax in which the curtain comes down on the NHS in financial flames". Instead he says there is "no *gotterdammerung*—but a final anticlimax as the firemen led by . . . the secretary of state rush onto the stage to douse the fire with buckets of money in the last act". He wrote that describing the NHS of the 1980s, but it is no less true of the NHS of the 1990s.[20] On 31 May 1998 the newspapers reported that the Government was about to announce a £12 billion injection of cash for the Health Service and for education but that the exact timing of the announcement would depend on England's performance in the World Cup. The chancellor did not want the good news submerged by a good soccer result or a bad result! Thus are we governed.

5.2.7 PFI

The recent, very public, twist to this tale of funding the Health Service is the continuing saga of PFI, the Private Finance Initiative. This is an initiative not solely directed at changing the way NHS capital projects are funded but is also being applied throughout the public services. The thesis, simplified, goes like this. We need a new hospital/hospital building, etc. We do not have the capital and we know that even if we did we are inefficient at arranging for buildings to go up to budget and on time. So let's get the more efficient private sector to put up the building, service it and have a lease on it. We will just pay them annually for the use of that resource or even better will give them our spare land or buildings in exchange and/or let them provide the support services that are needed in the hospital. All the Health Service now has to do is rent space for our doctors and nurses to treat patients in. It is much more complicated than that, of course, but the underlying thesis seemed sound and there was the encouraging prospect of consortia of financiers, builders and service specialists working together to do their own things well for the NHS.

Unfortunately, the process has been fraught with difficulties, many of which are complex but all of which have conspired to prevent the majority of projects going ahead. Five examples will suffice:

(1) *Scale.* Overall there were too many schemes. The initiative was intended to "let a thousand flowers bloom" but, of course, capital and backers and those capable of delivering were limited, so the number of projects has been curtailed. The scale of the projects' costs has escalated and analysis shows that in many instances the cost of achieving the objective using public money would have been less than if it was left to PFI consortia. Gaffney and Pollock studied 14 such projects and found that during development the estimated cost of the schemes rose by an average of 72%.[21]

(2) *Unrealistic expectations of performance.* Efficiency savings are often required in the use of the new buildings if the package is to be affordable, but these savings are often untested or unachievable. The Edinburgh Scheme, for example, expects a 35% increase in patient throughput per bed.

(3) *Risk transfer.* Risk transfer was inherent in the original PFI concept. The consortia would, in theory, carry part of the risk of future changes in work patterns, care purchasing, building regulations, etc. The consortia have, however, rather belatedly realised that almost all these issues are under government control and that therefore the government should bear more of the risk. This, known as the "ultra vires" issue, remains to be resolved, even though the NHS Private Finance Act of 1997 directly addressed it.

(4) *There is no such thing as free money.* All PFI projects are an impending debt on the public purse merely deferring current capital expenditure and replacing it by an increased current expenditure bill in the future; yet the Accounting Standards Board has been unable thus far to persuade the Treasury that these PFI projects need to be included in the PSBR (Public Sector Borrowing Requirement).

(5) *Employee considerations.* One of the factors inherent in most PFI schemes is the provision of non-clinical labour by the PFI partner. In many instances this may simply involve transferring the lowest paid NHS employees to a different employer potentially for a lower wage or into different conditions of employment. The unions regard this, of course, with considerable suspicion and the process has been bedevilled by uncertainty about "TUPE" (the Transfer of Undertakings [Protection of Employment]) where even European court rulings remain, as yet, unclear.

These and other problems lead one to consider whether PFI is really as good as once we thought. Is the need to get the right return on the capital really the right planning motive for the NHS and anyway can we really afford the uncertain future costs of PFI? There is after all, as the man said, "no such thing as a free lunch". The medical manager caught up in all this needs to remain very sanguine and not to get too carried away by the exciting prospect of a seemingly free new hospital!

5.3 Top to bottom: management structures and how they work

To the newcomer there is often confusion about who does what in the hierarchy of the NHS, who is accountable to whom. It is a topic where clear definitions are rare and where the actual dynamics only rarely reflect the ideal. In essence the NHS tree grows like this:

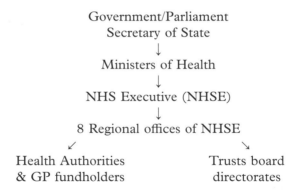

Government/Parliament
Secretary of State
↓
Ministers of Health
↓
NHS Executive (NHSE)
↓
8 Regional offices of NHSE
↙ ↘
Health Authorities   Trusts board
& GP fundholders   directorates

This is very simplified. There are for instance other agencies such as the Medicines Control Agency which are directly controlled by the Department of Health. Additionally there are multitudinous side branches adorned with advisory bodies and think tanks, professional panels, steering groups, liaison committees, focus groups and advisors, but for all this there is fundamentally a straightline chain of responsibility between the individual doctor and the Secretary of State. When the reforms were put in place that set up NHS trusts there was an expectation that there would be significant independence for trusts from the previous hierarchical controls. In reality no great differences were encountered.

176

Outside the hospital trusts there is a reconfiguration of primary care and purchasing authorities underway at the time of writing to establish "Primary Care Groups".

5.3.1 Ministers

The Secretary of State is responsible to Parliament for the functions and functioning of the NHS. To assist him in this he has ministers, currently two. These are of lower profile and have specific areas of concern. One of the two ministers is currently responsible for women's issues. Although the Secretary of State and ministers are advised by the Department of Health, the NHS Executive and the Chief Medical Officer, they are politicians and their horizons rarely extend beyond the next election. Also, because their concerns come to us through the distorting lens of the media we tend to hear their views crudely put. As a medical manager struggling to get things done, it is easy to be upset by the pronouncements of ministers; we should not be, they are not intended for us. There is often, however, a streak of more than just performance art in the minister's show; there may truly be some self delusion. Amanda Mitchison commented at the end of her interview with Baroness Jay, Minister of Health in the Lords:[22]

> we seem to have been talking about two quite different health services. The NHS you and I know is a place of crumbling buildings, and long waits, and understaffing, and bureaucracies busy robbing Peter to just about pay Paul—and yet, for all that, it still remains, on the whole, pretty good. The grot is just part of the British experience ... An undeniable fact of existence. But not in Margaret Jay's book. Her hospitals are brimming with eager beavers and exciting initiatives and optimistic, can-do martinets on greater efficiency drives. This is the world as presented so often to us by politicians, limitless possibilities on no more cash. Never acknowledge, never concede, refute the irrefutable. They must take us for such fools.

In July 1998 Baroness Jay was promoted to full cabinet rank.

Do not worry. What really matters is that the advice ministers get is as sound as possible and that in your turn you listen only to what is actually planned to happen; that will be finalised not in Westminster but will emerge as papers from the NHS Executive in Leeds, distilled as another ubiquitous Executive Letter or Health

Service Circular. If you are in management long enough, you will be able to enjoy the hobby of matching circulars that reflect in a deadpan way governments' about turns. Competition one year, cooperation the next, care in the community one year, care in hospital another.

The Department of Health, by the way, is not unaudited. The Public Accounts Committee and the Audit Commission and of course the Treasury keep a beady and possibly jaundiced eye on it. There is also the Health Service Commissioner or Ombudsman to watch out for "maladministration", of whom more in Section 6.9. The Department of Health is the rump of the old career-based civil service that advised and transmitted instructions for implementation but had little interest in finance or direct management. Following the Fulton Committee Report in 1968 this began to change and eventually that change delivered the separation of the managerial arm as the NHS Management Executive.

5.3.2 The Chief Medical Officer

The Chief Medical Officer (CMO) is a high profile job and doctors often ask where this post fits into the management hierarchy. The CMO is not in the managerial chain but is the medical senior advisor to the Secretary of State as well as other government bodies. The CMO is effectively the Director of Public Health for England. That the last CMO, Sir Kenneth Calman, has his name attached to two initiatives, the "Calmanisation" of training and the Calman–Hine proposals for cancer services, illustrates the centrality of the role in planning, although recent reductions in the CMO's staff and the invention of the NHS Executive by the last government has reduced the CMO's powers. The CMO's responsibilities may be summarised as follows:

- Monitor the state of the public's health and evaluate the influences on it.
- Ensure high-quality input is available for the formation and implementation of policy and for issues affecting health services generally.
- Maintain effective links with other government departments on all questions affecting the public's health.

- Maintain effective links between the Government and the medical profession.
- Ensure the UK is represented on medical matters internationally.
- The CMO also sits on a number of bodies such as the Medical Research Council and the General Medical Council.

5.3.3 The NHS Executive and regional offices[23]

The NHS Executive consists of the headquarters in Leeds and eight regional offices that were established when the old regional health authorities were abolished in 1994. Headquarters is responsible for:

- Leading strategic and policy developments.
- Securing and allocating financial resources.
- Supporting the Minister in accounting for the use of those resources.
- Setting the framework for performance management.
- Developing national policies on manpower and its training.
- Developing and evaluating a strategy for implementing evidence-based healthcare.
- Developing and evaluating the NHS Research and Development Strategy.

The regional offices
These have a more practical managerial role in that they:

- Are responsible for overseeing the purchasing functions within their regions.
- Monitor the financial performance of trusts and also their performance in a limited number of non-financial areas.
- Manage the performance of health authorities including their compliance with ministers' policies. (It is worth noting that this broad remit does not also apply in their relationship with trusts.)
- Prioritise and approve capital allocation and capital projects.
- Liaise with universities in relation to medical and dental education. The regional postgraduate dean's office is a part of the NHS Executive regional office.
- Set the regional research and development agenda.
- Plan the regional workforce.
- Establish community health councils.

- Develop public health locally.
- Dispose of redundant properties.

The NHS Executive is managerially an arm of the NHS rather than a part of the traditional Whitehall orientated Civil Service. It is staffed largely by people who have had front-line NHS managerial experience.

5.3.4 Trust structures

There is of course more to the NHS than trusts, but a description of trusts will serve to illustrate typical mechanics. We have already seen that there are usually three tiers of management in trusts, a board, an executive group, both of which are responsible for the whole organisation, and below that subgroupings typically called clinical directorates, which manage the day-to-day business of particular services, surgery, pathology, critical care, whatever.

The board

The trust board mimics to some extent the board of any commercial company, with its chairman, non-executive directors (NEDs) and executive members. The board of an NHS Trust is a statutory body with its membership pre-figured. There is a chairman, appointed by the Secretary of State. He is usually a lay person but with some experience of the Health Service, as well as the running of an organisation. Next there are NEDs, normally four to six; they are lay people and if the trust is a teaching one, one NED will normally be a university representative such as the dean of the medical school. The NEDs are appointed by the Secretary of State, with advice of course. Politicised commentators rail against this as another example of lack of democracy, deriding them as "ministerial stooges"[24] but in truth the NHS is an organ of a democratically elected government, so a separate democratic process for the selection of board members is not the issue, it is the ability of boards to judge and reflect the wishes and needs of the public that is the issue.

After the NEDs there are the executive members. The chief executive, medical director, the directors of nursing, of finance and of personnel. There may be a few others, but normally these others are non-clinical senior managers, for example a chief operating officer, a director of strategy. The medical director and the director of nursing, and occasionally a dean, are the only people with any direct clinical experience on the board. The functions of executive members are clear from their titles, though they take joint responsibility for board decisions. The board as a whole essentially has five responsibilities:

- To set the strategic direction of the organisation within the overall policies and priorities of the Government and the NHS Executive.
- To oversee the delivery of planned results.
- To ensure effective financial stewardship and value for money.
- To ensure that high standards of corporate governance and personal behaviour are maintained.
- To ensure that there is effective dialogue between the organisation and the local community on its plans and performance.

Beyond that the chairman and non-executives have a role in the appointment, review and remuneration of the chief executive and other executive directors.[25]

Non-executive board members typically have a special interest in one or more of these areas depending on their expertise. It's tough being an NED. It's time consuming and most spend more time on it than the stipulated 20 days per year (the average is 34). It is difficult to be grafted onto an industry about which you may know little or nothing. Surveys have shown that the main activity of NEDs is simply querying and probing of executive decisions, when in theory they should be more directly involved with the strategic decision making and option appraisal. Unfortunately NEDs tend to be quickly overloaded with the unimaginative chores of disciplinary and grievance hearings, appointment on appeal panels and independent panels dealing with complaints. The net result is that the NHS NEDs do more than their private sector equivalents yet have difficulty focusing on the real problems in the organisation. During the last Conservative government, NEDs tended to come from commercial backgrounds and were able reasonably quickly to come to grips with the business aspects of board activities. The new government has purged 75% of these posts, the holders of which were thought to be politically unacceptable and not sensitive enough to the views of the local populace. Newer appointees are in theory made as a result of a more open process. Much was made of equality but, worryingly, the political allegiance of applicants has to be declared in advance.

By 5 February 1998, 886 new NEDs had been appointed. The ethnic minority representation has been corrected, it is now 9%, which exceeds the 7% in the population as a whole. By 31 May 1998 36% of chairpersons and 52% of NEDs were women. Of those NEDs who said they were politically active, the overwhelming majority were Labour supporters, these included 111 Labour local councillors. Let us hope that, whatever their politics, closer links to the community of the new NEDs will make for a more constructive dialogue between trusts and the communities they serve and that they will be sympathetic to the social audit side of a board's business, defining and auditing the trust's moral and social responsibilities to all the stakeholders, community, patients, and staff.

Whatever the future, I will guarantee that at the moment 90% of the members of staff of any trust you care to name do not know the names or the faces of their NEDs.

Much effort is put into improving the performance of boards, but many of the lists of tasks and developments needed are daunting to the point of unachievability.[26] The anxiety is that the really talented and experienced people that the NHS needs will be put off by the unrewarding and unstimulating chores that can characterise an NED's time in the NHS.

Members of a trust board carry legal responsibilities both corporately and personally, and The Treasury Solicitor's Department has recently highlighted the adequacy of the insurance cover currently available for them so new members should check that there is appropriate insurance cover to protect them.

Clinical directors and executive groups

Boards meet on average once a month, perhaps for 3 hours; not long enough to manage a hospital trust, it's merely the captain's bridge. For day-to-day management, for the generation of new proposals and the solution of current problems, the engine room of any trust is the executive group. This comprises the executive members of the board i.e. the chief executive, the medical director, the director of finance, etc., but to be effective it will need to draw in the next layers of the NHS hierarchy—the clinical directors and the non-clinical managers. How best to do this is far from certain and the solutions vary from trust to trust. The commonest number of clinical directors in a trust is eight but a significant number have more than 20. In these trusts the problem is the same as throughout all organisations, how do you have an executive grouping small enough to be effective as a committee (5–15), yet not so small as to exclude the crucial range of opinion and expertise? Clinical directors can be a trifle prima donna-ish, and even paranoid if they feel excluded. They tend to feel that the specialty they lead is so important that it needs its own seat on the top table. But in almost all trusts there are too many of them to be in an executive group, so they need themselves to be grouped with an appointed or elected leader sitting on the executive, or else they need their own "parliament" which elects a few of its number to participate in the executive.

Whatever solution you use to bind in the clinical directors there is another problem, that of the non-clinical senior managers. So keen has the NHS been to involve doctors in management that clinical directors have been given a sort of spurious seniority in the system, they do after all have no real claim to senior management posts in that they have no special training or experience and many have no particular aptitude for it. Nor in an egalitarian health service do they have any moral right to be occupying most of the seats at the top table—it's an accident of history. An accident that leaves the non-clinical senior managers sometimes relegated to a major domo, adjutant, aide-de-camp or head butler role. For some no doubt that is promotion beyond their competence, but for many it is demeaning and inappropriate, so they too need to be swept up into the senior executive group. If this is not done, the danger is that they will establish a parallel network of opinion and decision taking, alongside the clinical director to chief executive axis.

The next contentious issue to be resolved is whether the chairman of the hospital medical committee should have a seat on the executive. The members of the executive should be cabinet members sharing the decision making, so in theory there is no place for an "outsider" who may have a different agenda. The decision probably ought to be an individual one for each trust, depending on the character of the person involved.

5.3.5 A senior cadre

An innovative way of tying in both the clinical and non-clinical members, and others central to the working of a large organisation, is deliberately to establish a defined senior group, an officer class described in my trust with redolences of lost communism as "the senior cadre". The group meets together, debates together and is briefed together preferentially within the organisation. The senior cadre posts are graded and the grading goes with the job and with competencies, but the cadre allows egalitarian team working as all are valued equally and can in theory progress to any other senior cadre post. It has the added advantage of addressing the neglected problem of succession planning. The only downside is that it can allow the next layer down to feel disenfranchised and can limit new blood reaching jobs that fall vacant. On balance, however, it seems to work well.

References

1 Eco U. *The Name of the Rose*. Minerva, 1992, p. 218.
2 Harrison S, Hunter DJ, Pollitt C. *The Dynamics of British Health Policy*. London: Unwin Hyman, 1990, p. 2.
3 Rein M. *Social Science and Public Policy*. London: Penguin, 1976, p. 103. Quoted by Allsop J. *Health Policy and the National Health*. London: Longman, 1984.
4 Harrison S, Hunter DJ, Pollitt C. *The Dynamics of British Health Policy*. London: Unwin Hyman, 1990, pp. 6–8.
5 Secretaries of State for Health. *Working for Patients*. Cmnd 555. London: HMSO, 1992, p. 119.
6 Butler J. *Patients, Policies and Politics*. Milton Keynes, Buckinghamshire: Open University Press, 1992, p. 119.
7 Webster C. *The National Health Service, a Political History*. Oxford: Oxford University Press, 1998, p. 203.
8 Soderlund N *et al.* Impact of NHS reforms on English hospital productivity: analysis of the first three years. *Br Med J* 1997;**315**: 1126–9.
9 Oakley A. In: Oakley A, Williams AS, eds. *The Politics of the Welfare State*. London: UCL Press, 1994, pp. 1–17.
10 Dunleavy P, O'Leary B. *Theories of the State; the politics of liberal democracy*. London: Macmillan, 1987, pp. 193–7.
11 Griffiths R (Chairman). *Report of the NHS Management Enquiry*. London: DHSS, 1983.
12 Gray A, Jenkins B. Public management and the National Health Service. In: *Managing Health Care: challenges for the 90s*. London: Saunders, 1995, pp. 4–32.
13 Jenkins S. *Accountable to None: the Tory nationalisation of Britain*. London: Hamish Hamilton, 1995.
14 Klein R. *The Politics of the National Health Service*, 2nd edn. London: Longman, 1989.
15 Bryson B. *Notes From a Small Island*. London: Secker & Warburg, 1996.
16 Office of Health Economics figures cited in *Br Med J* 1967;**315**:568.
17 Sheldon TA. Formula fever; allocating resources in the NHS. *Br Med J* 1997;**315**:964.

18 Getzen TE. *Health Economics: fundamentals and flow of funds.* New York: Wiley, 1997, p. 442.
19 Newchurch Health Briefing. *Strategic Changes in the NHS.* 3, 1996.
20 Klein R. *The Politics of the NHS*, 2nd edn. London: Longman, 1989.
21 Price D. Profiting from closure: the private finance initiative and the NHS. *Br Med J* 1997;**315**:1479–80.
22 Mitchison AA. Picture of perfection. *The Sunday Telegraph Magazine* 1998;15 February: 14.
23 Ham C. The organisation of the NHS. In: *The 1998/99 NHS Handbook.* London: NAHAT, Macmillan, 1998.
24 Webster C. *The National Health Service, a Political History.* Oxford: Oxford University Press, 1998.
25 NAHAT. *Up-date* 1996;14 April.
26 The Audit Commission. *Taken on Board.* London: HMSO, 1995.

6 Special Problems

6.1 CHANGE

This chapter outlines some personal views about the options that clinicians/directors have in handling change. If anyone doubts the quantity and magnitude of changes engulfing the Health Service in the UK, they need only to weigh their non-clinical mail or review the recent year's outpouring of executive letters from the NHS Executive. At the time of writing there are literally dozens of "initiatives" (an Orwellian misnomer!) underway with central "guidance".

Change has always been inherent in the business of medicine, but it comes in fits and starts and we are currently in the middle of a full-blown, rather protracted grand mal fit. This discomforts everyone, for it disturbs their lives and the framework that makes their lives neat and comprehensible.

Ubi stabilitas ibi religio

Where there is stability there is faith

But without change there is no progress; though of course change *ipso facto* does not imply progress. The most taxing task in the business of management is the management of change, for change is the bedfellow of conflict and of stress. In dealing with the topic it is worth splitting it up into three:

(1) Your personal position in relationship to change.
(2) Implementing change in the organisation.
(3) Responding to change by influencing upwards in the organisation.

6.1.1 Personal response to change

The changes that tax you most are invariably of someone else's making and their implementation may or may not be to your taste. Indeed you would be an unimaginative and uneducated clinician

186

if you had no views about the ideas behind any change. I suppose there are some bureaucrats who are content to act merely as a passive channel for change, a kind of crustacean effector arm. Doctors do not fit this niche in nature's hierarchy and there's the problem for you the clinician and you the manager. Firstly it's important to get things straight about a medical manager's place in the process of managing change. For most clinicians caught up in the process of managing healthcare the changes that affect them are imposed from outside their own areas in the organisation and usually from outside the patch within which they have their regular communications and working relationships. "Outside" being government, NHS Executive, regional organisations, purchasers, royal colleges and a host of other bureaucracies interested in the exercise of power without the tiresome practical difficulties of implementing their new ideas. Before you, the poor manager, try to implement someone else's bright ideas a moment's self analysis is worthwhile to review your place in "the change process". For my own part I am a natural conservative, liturgically I prefer Gregorian chant and guttering candles to happy-clappy guitarists and television lights, but then that is romanticism. The chanting monk is probably tuberculous and his congregation starving, whereas the happy-clappy goes home in her car to a hot lunch . . . So what is that about self analysis? Simply this. If you have an instinct to resist change think the problems through intellectually, critically read the views of others including BMJ editorials, glossy government hand-outs and newspaper comment, and decide whether you are whole-heartedly in support of change or at least acquiescent. Conversely if you find the business of change stimulating and the rollercoaster of making it happen exciting, then look into your soul—or rather your physiology—to check that you are not just getting a buzz out of the adrenaline. That done the old reactionary or the young revolutionary can place himself in relation to the change. If he disagrees with it for good objective reasons that he can support in debate, then he should object in the right forum. If he still objects after the debate then he should resign or swallow his pride and do the best he can to implement the change without spending time denying its value to all and sundry.

That is all very simple, reality is usually more difficult. Take the "New Deal" for example. Many of us feel deeply unhappy about it for reasons we can argue; it erodes the vocational thread that should imbue a career in medicine, and in practical terms it can interfere with the continuity of patient care and the education of young doctors. But it is the law (even European law is law!). Most junior doctors want it and perhaps the drawbacks can be overcome; so let's support it while trying to ameliorate the problems it generates.

The response of individuals and groups to change usually follows this pattern! (Figure 6.1):

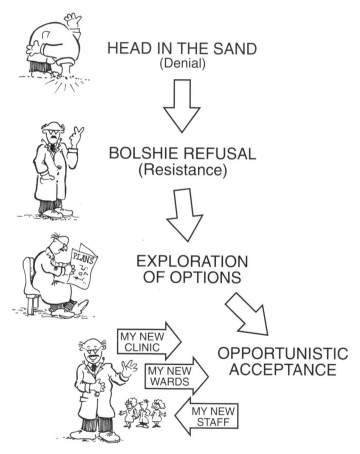

Figure 6.1   Responses to change.

While your self respect will demand that you continue to comment *upwards* (see below) and at executive level on changes you think inappropriate, you must be consistent when working towards achieving them. This is not simply a matter of cabinet responsibility, it is a practical matter of being credible as a manager. Effective implementation does not mean you have to deny problems. It is a matter of how you do it and the most important thing is that whoever you are leading should not be confused by your actions, wondering if you really want them to implement the change or not.

6.1.2 Implementing change

Nothing would ever be attempted if all possible objections must first be overcome (SAM JOHNSON)

The actual process of planning change needs to be handled in a cool, sequential way. There will be plenty of room for gesture and intuition in the day-to-day hurly-burly of implementation. The important first step is a careful overview to:

(1) *Define the change and prioritise it* among other changes that are planned.
(2) *Identify the effects the change will have* on the people, on the organisation as a whole and on the functions of its departments. Make sure you know all the ramifications of the change you propose. How many people and actions will this change effect? Did you realise that moving ENT from one hospital to another affects the day-to-day management of stroke victims because the speech therapy department will need to move too? Did you know that removing children's services from one hospital to another may lose your anaesthetic department its educational recognition? Now re-visit the change and decide if you still want to make it. If you do, make a preliminary assessment of the steps needed to achieve the change. This must be done in consultation with those who will be affected.
(3) If having looked at the details you still plan to go ahead, *communicate the changes* openly, honestly and widely remembering that those who oppose change often do so late and affect not to have been told about it earlier. Consultants, in particular, sometimes give the impression that if they have not been informed verbally and personally then they could not be expected to know about change. Some major changes require

formal public consultation especially if services are to be removed from one hospital to another. This is a time consuming and difficult process and will need to be orchestrated by an outside agency, usually the local purchasing authority.

(4) *Do not overstate or misrepresent* the benefits of the change you plan. Audiences are sophisticated about the implications of change; indeed they might be more sophisticated than you.

(5) *Re-appraise the project* yet again in the light of the feedback you have had from the communication exercise. This is particularly important because there are often knock-on effects from a change which are not immediately apparent or are minimised by the enthusiasts who want the change. Very few changes are universally welcomed; thus the difficult part of the process is often to hold firm where there are a large number of opponents yet the bulk of the evidence suggests that the change is necessary and beneficial.

Once you have clearly embarked on the process of change opponents may start to use alternative channels to prevent the change. They will appeal over your head to more senior people within the organisation. They will appeal outside the organisation. They will try to sway those who previously supported the change and if they feel passionately about it they will not be beyond dirty tricks, misinformation and disinformation; hence the importance of the next phase.

(6) *Commitment planning.* The neat concept described by Barnes[1] requires an analysis of who in the organisation needs to be committed to the change, what role they need to play, where they stand now and how they need to change if things are to happen smoothly. Barnes identifies four categories of commitment for the key players:

"*No Commitment*"—likely to oppose the change.
"*Let It Happen*"—will not oppose the initiative but will not actively support it.
"*Help It Happen*"—must provide resources (time or equipment).
"*Make It Happen*"—must be actively involved and willing to lead.

He suggests that this exercise is done formally and the positions of the key players tabulated (Figure 6.2).

Key players	No commitment	Let it happen	Help it happen	Make it happen
Chief executive officer				OX
Chairman St Judes medical staff committee	O ⟶	X		
UMB member A		O ⟶		X
UMB member B			O ⟶	X
Consultant C		O ⟶ X		
Consultant D		X ⟵		O
Manager E		O ⟶		X

O=present position; X=required position.
(Consultant D has poor interpersonal skills and his enthusiasm is likely to be counter-productive)

Figure 6.2 Charting personal commitment to change. (Reproduced with permission from: Simpson and Smith, *Management for Doctors.* London: BMJ Books, 1995.)

(7) *Action planning.* Having gathered all views on the original proposal, sifted them, rejected some and incorporated some, it is time formally to list all the actions needed to reach the goal. Some of these will be on the critical path i.e. if they don't happen or don't happen on time everything else is held up. In most projects it helps to construct a Gantt chart (Figure 6.3). This is easy for most of those involved to understand and helps to focus everyone's minds on the "choke points" in the implementation process.

I have carefully not called this stage the "business planning stage", though the elements of a business plan will need to

191

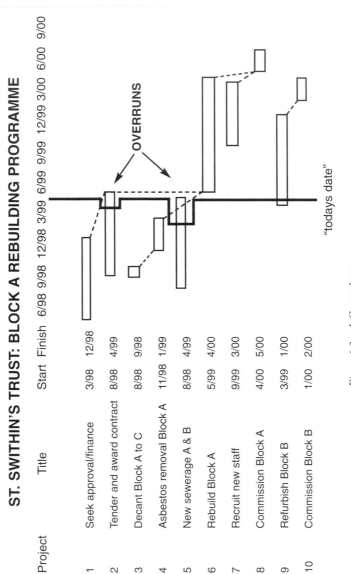

Figure 6.3 A Gantt chart

be there identifying the targets, the route, the resources to be used, the cost and the benefits versus the disbenefits. However a too formal business planning process has in my experience a deadening, even stupefying effect and can be totally counter-productive if teams are expected to produce a watertight, polished plan relating to something fluid and evolving.

It is, however, critical at this stage to identify which staff will be involved in making change happen and whether extra resources are needed. Taking staff away from their normal roles can be disruptive, and the ill effects of this are quickly used by detractors further to pillory the process and those involved. Having identified staff it is important to identify a *project manager* even for a small project who can be set a target and timetable.

(8) *Re-appraisal.* Having followed through steps (1) to (7), re-visit the concept which has set the change process in motion. Does it still make sense? Can you still afford it? Will it achieve what you want? Detailed honest planning often shows up a need for more personnel and resources than you had at first thought, so decide if you still wish to go ahead or whether you could better put the effort to something else on your list of priorities. To conclude that it is "too much hassle for too little gain" is a perfectly honourable conclusion and not going ahead is not necessarily a sign of managerial weakness.

(9) *Re-communicate.* Yes, we are going ahead and here's the plan.

(10) *Go for it!* Projects that limp along slowly demoralise everyone. Money, staff and enthusiasm leach away into more achievable ends and managerial credibility is lost. Delaying because of quibbles over cost is common. Quibbles about small, over-budget items tend to be counter-productive because the delay and extra work that is incurred have a habit of costing more than the quibble would have saved.

During the implementation keep the troops informed especially about problems. One of the most successful projects I have watched underway carried everyone along with it because the architects drawings were attached to the walls, the work could be seen progressing, the stage in the timetable and the problems with the project were all honestly and briefly annotated and stuck up as wall posters from day to day.

(11) Lastly, do not forget that the completion of a change project, whether it be new procedures, a new building or the start-up

of a new service, requires major commitment to *training and induction* for all those involved. Too often a budget is not set aside for this nor time.

(12) When the project is complete and successful *announce it, be proud about it* and make sure you thank all those whose hard work might otherwise go unrecognised.

6.1.3 Managing responses upwards

"Managing up" is the business of influencing the organisational levels above you so as to modulate if necessary the projects they are asking you to implement. It covers everything from a response to a draft proposal from government to a frank workers' revolt. It is an important concept because the notion that "managing up" can and does occur goes a long way to alleviate the sense of powerlessness that so many in the Health Service feel. Given the enormous size of the NHS and the great distance between central decision-makers and the Health Service coalface, you would think that as a medical manager your options for influencing policy retroactively are small. This is not so. Regardless of the shifts towards deprofessionalisation and marginalisation of doctors that has occurred, they still nonetheless have the moral whiphand in most situations, and if they are honest and careful they can still be regarded as the arbiters of what is appropriate in healthcare.

The ways for doctors to "manage up" are multitudinous; some are proper and some are improper. As a clinician you can manage up by way of the BMA and its representatives or the royal colleges and their representatives. They both have ways into the decision-making processes. If you are a manager you can and should join the British Association of Medical Managers and if you are a medical director the Association of Trust Medical Directors. Occasionally you will get a chance to express a view to visiting dignitaries, chairs of health boards, MPs, junior ministers. If you really feel that is likely to be a useful channel you should carefully orchestrate your approach in advance and decide who says what and when. Passionate gripes over coffee are ill received; a quiet exposure to the practical aspects of the problem during the tour are more likely to be effective. A "memory bite" to match the politicians "sound bite".

The problem about professional organisations as formal channels for "managing up" when change is afoot is that although government "initiatives" are sent out for consultation, the timescale for these "consultation exercises" is, either through incompetence or design, so short as to make a considered view difficult and a properly researched one impossible. The BMA is often given only a few weeks in which to reply, while those of us further down the heap will often receive our papers after the date for receipt of replies. So not surprisingly other ways of getting heard are forced upon us.

Your next weapon is formal letters to policy makers, solicited or unsolicited. These need careful handling. Non-clinical managers are always amazed at doctors' preference for writing letters rather than making face-to-face contact but that's the way we do things and in many contexts the good letter is effective. The angry/outraged/passionate letter is all very well but remember always:

(1) Sleep on what you have written before sending it.
(2) Share it with another person before you send it.
(3) Get your facts right!

Even if your letter is nine-tenths right it will be tarnished by wrong facts or assumptions. Even a wrong paragraph will tarnish a whole letter and allow the minister's aide with a smile to fold it neatly into a paper dart and launch it at the wastepaper basket.

Oh, and by the way, don't send out too many copies. I have seen letters of the most trivial nature copied to the Prime Minister, the Secretary of State, the presidents of all the royal colleges, etc., etc. By all means copy but try to pick the people who are likely to see it and whose actions are genuinely likely to be changed by your letter.

Next, the most dangerous option of all, the media.

The media

I mention this here to dismiss it as a proper means of managing up. It is useful to believe that the press is a whore pretending to please but intent only on its own profit. The information it uses is usually unvalidated, biased and inconsistent; its use of that information cynical. At the top of the broadsheet tree it makes some efforts to be responsible (though less effort to be accurate) and at the bottom of the tabloid tree it makes efforts only to amaze, alarm, titivate or amuse. Your own attempts at forcing change on an unwilling government or the disgruntled doctor's attempts to change the plans your trust has carefully construed are all grist to the mill when seen from the press's point of view. They'll believe what you tell them, flatter and cajole you into saying more than you should, and in a day they will be gone, your passionate concerns turned into chip wrappings. All personal relations with the media risk bringing out your worst streaks of vanity, and appearance on the television verges on reckless self exposure as all your normal reflexes towards caution and balance are abandoned.

It's not all true of course but if you believe that it's almost true it may help you to keep out of trouble. If you must deal with the media do so through or with the advice of a professional public relations officer. If having to deal with the media is a habit then go on a course to learn how to do it safely.

6.1.4 Types of change

The sort of changes that will impact on you could be categorised in five ways:

(1) Ideological change—political change, e.g. fundholding general practices.
(2) Legislative change, e.g. changes in employment legislation.
(3) Functional change—the managerial meat, e.g. service reconfigurations, mergers, enlarging, shrinking, etc.
(4) Technical change due to advances in medical care, e.g. setting up non-invasive surgery.
(5) Fatuous change. These changes may not in themselves be inappropriate or harmful but are those embarked on for cosmetic or fashion reasons, e.g. changing the logo on the notepaper.

Another categorisation of change is simply to divide it into big projects and little projects. Big projects such as "Calman" or the "New Deal" are those where the end point is defined but the mechanics of getting there are not always clear and the funding almost invariably absent. It is these sort of projects that have the greater power to demotivate and demoralise teams. The little projects, by contrast, if well done and funded tend to be achievable and achieved and give all those involved a sense of satisfaction. Small is beautiful!

6.1.5 Incremental change and large projects

Because of the difficulties of large projects their achievement needs to be divided up very carefully into bite-sized pieces at the outset.

This particularly involves the setting of realistic targets. One of the most irritating features of the original implementation schemes for the "New Deal" was the assumption that everything would be achieved within a very short timespan. This was impossible for managers on the ground and led merely to confrontation between visiting teams and the managers who had not achieved and between the managers who were not achieving and the clinicians who could not continue to deliver a service if the changes were imposed quickly. New managers have a habit of wanting the shiny, full-built end product quickly and may need to be reminded that this is not always the appropriate way forward. One new postgraduate dean had to be taken aside and told "you have too many objectives that require explicit action". That sounds Byzantine but was at least pragmatic. The same postgraduate dean told me that dealing with the almost unachievable big projects which were required of him was like banging his head against jelly; all the frustrations but none of the relieving pleasure of pain that he would have had if it had been a wall.

6.1.6 Small change projects

People will commit an enormous amount of effort to small local projects, an extension to a ward, a new ITU system, a refurbished clinic, a new piece of technology, a new way of running a clinic, a new way of delivering education. As a medical manager or member of an executive group, you will be brought many of these proposals and your wish to be positive and supportive needs to be tempered by some practicalities. You might usefully ask the following questions of the project:

- Is it really needed?
- Is it thought through?
- Is it properly costed?
- Are the knock-on effects on other specialties or areas understood?
- Will it fly? That is can it be funded? Does it rely on the enthusiasm of only one person? Is there space?
- What will happen down the line 1–5 years from now?
- How does it fit in with the institution's overall needs and plans?

As a medical manager or member of a committee you have useful experience which can be brought to bear on the critical appraisal of such proposals. You can protect the organisation from:

- Zany ideas.
- Overbidding.
- Shroud waving.
- Undeclared effects on other departments.

After a while you become sensitive to the ploys which enthusiastic, well-meaning clinicians bring to bear on the presentation of their pet projects. The standard bidding ploys include:

(1) "It will bring in extra money" (*your response*: "prove it, is the money out there?").
(2) "If we don't have it we will not be recognised as a serious unit/by the SAC/for university training" (*your response*: "who said so? when was a unit last derecognised for not having this?").
(3) "If we don't have it patients will suffer" (*your response*: "how? how much? how many? prove it!").
(4) "If we don't have it we cannot recruit/retain staff" (*your response*: "what is your current staff turnover? what evidence do you have that the absence of this is losing you staff?").

Of course you must not just baldly recite this Killjoy's catechism, your normal tone will naturally be positive and encouraging, avoiding the traditional "The answer's NO! now what's the question?".

6.1.7 Project overload

For the upper echelons of management there is a tendency to commission or embrace more and more projects. The changes in the environment around seem to dictate it and not to respond implies that you are unaware of the "climate of change" and indeed that if you are not responding you are not managing in all senses of the word; so the upper echelons of management have a reprehensible habit of passing on all these initiatives half digested to the middle and lower grade managers and their clinical colleagues. And why not? The cynic would say that the initiators don't have to do the work, the middle managers who work through the project don't mind, if they did their *raison d'être* would evaporate. Middle managers don't mind, why would they because the chore, the leg work requires effort not by them but by subcommittees, doctors, nurses, physiotherapists, secretaries and others further down in the organisation, so what's the problem? The problem is one of overload.

Overload is tolerated by the workers when it is judged to be appropriate. Doctors and nurses will work endlessly when patients' needs are the imperative. Junior managers will work to open a ward or deal with a backlog, but when a project is not understood or not agreed upon by the do-ers then it will not happen. This is a major problem in the Health Service where so many "initiatives" are seen as superfluous to the core business of healthcare. The argument that the latest initiative is just to tidy up the remaining loose ends does not ring true either. The "last push" is seen by most clinicians in the same light as a subaltern's in the First World War ordered to make "the final push", rather than the midwife urging a final push when all but the baby's legs are in view. How do we control the flow of projects? Essentially it is a matter of "managing up" which was described earlier, something of which boards, executives and senior managers do too little and to which the NHS Executive and regions and colleges are too impervious. It would be nice if there were coupons or some form of rationing for the NHS Executive. If it was only allowed five new initiatives a year it might think through the ones it proposed a little more carefully and spend more time on less projects, rather than inadequate time on a large number. The Executive, in common with all other layers of senior management, needs three virtues when looking at a project, *insight, humility* and *a willingness to consult*, and should always consider before starting a new initiative whether or not the managerial effort might not be better spent in ensuring that the last project commissioned had actually happened and was having the intended effect. Senior managers in the Health Service intent on radical change might usefully read Hobsbawm on the French Revolution. He observed that it succeeded because the changes were formalised by philosophers into an intellectually coherent set of plans, and were effective because they genuinely reflected the people's needs. The people could focus on the reasons for their dissent and could understand and support each solution at a personal level, whether it was land reform, reduced taxation, fair local administration or whatever. So many of the changes forced onto the Health Service fail because they have not been formalised in an intellectually or economically sustainable way and are couched in such a way that the ordinary peasants working in the Health Service have difficulty perceiving them to be of personal relevance.

6.2 RATIONALISATIONS AND MERGERS

Hardly a day goes by without a public proposal for the merger of departments or of hospitals or the transfer of a service from one organisation to another. The proposals are usually made on the basis that this will provide the population with a better and more efficient service, although in truth the proposal is usually made primarily for financial reasons although sometimes mergers are needed to weld critically small units into larger, viable ones to satisfy the needs of providing an increasingly hyper-specialised service, to provide a mass of staff of sufficient size to be recognised for training or quite simply to resolve the hours of work issues inherent in the New Deal and Calman proposals for training.

6.2.1 The stress of mergers

It is a fact of life that Nature is red in tooth and claw and large animals eat smaller ones. So with mergers. The naturally predatory behaviour of all organisations leads them to enjoy colonisations, which sounds unkind but is true. Nine times out of ten there are winners, and winners enjoy being winners, and of course losers hate being losers; all of this generates a lot of *angst* but does not slow the process too much. Mergers where the two parties are of equal sizes carry the most difficulties. For example the merger of Guy's and St Thomas' Hospitals was, and remains, agonisingly difficult in its everyday expression. Both hospitals were of the same size, same budget, same fame (each, of course, would dispute that) and had the same sized power base, but were culturally different. The decision as to the dominant partner in a geographical sense was decided on data that could (but not necessarily should) have been argued to the opposite conclusion. In fact, there was no very obvious winner and loser, both organisations won something and both lost something; but Guy's perceived itself the loser and the delicacy of the equation has goaded the Save Guy's Campaign and many people working within the organisation to subvert the process of merger in large or small ways. Whether that is an admirable commitment to a different vision or just short-sighted cussedness is a matter of opinion, but it certainly helps no one in the long run except some politicians. The situation in other balanced mergers is, I'm told, similar.

Could these, or any other mergers, have been managed differently? Looking back the answer is almost certainly a grudging "yes". A shorter timescale for the decision, a definite timescale for the grieving and then much more forceful efforts to get on with normal life would, undoubtedly, have improved the process for the participants. Doctors who spend their lives dealing with mortal illness ought to know about these things. However I confess that it was only in the midst of the Guy's & St Thomas' merger that I came to realise how like a death it seemed for many at Guy's, and how important is the management of the grieving, and how important to understand that the behaviour of some is very akin to that of those close to a dying person; inappropriately focused anger, denial, and inability to function effectively.

The arrangement of a merger between departments or hospitals taps into some of the deepest human feelings. Feelings about sacred places, tribal kinship, hierarchical status, and the responsibilities of a continuous lineage. These are feelings familiar and fascinating to the social anthropologist but a major problem for managers; so the first and crucial message about merger is to be very sensitive to those feelings, very wary of the trouble they will cause and very, very sure of the benefits that might accrue from merger. Has the team's morale been valued sufficiently? Will the benefits of merger be sufficient to justify the problems you are about to cause yourself and others? Which leads to the second message which is do not expect all the planned benefits of a merger actually to accrue. A certain overstatement of the benefits is necessary to energise the people involved but do not fool yourself that they'll happen. The Department of Health has claimed that each of the 16 mergers planned would produce minimum net savings of 8 million pounds in 2 years due to "reduced red tape". This is an assumption about the financial benefits of merger which has been well documented as being false both in the USA and the UK. It is against this background that managers should plan mergers. Non-clinical managers rarely understand the *volksgeist*, the cultural pride of the clinical teams involved, a feeling that may have built up over many years and have been reinforced by the clonal selection processes of generations of interview committees. When teams of different

201

cultures are merged, a lot of problems appear which would not have been predicted. Every little thing can cause trouble:

"We do it like this."

"Oh well, I am sorry but we do it like this."

Some people may make much of these differences further to discredit the merger. In other businesses and in industry, you simply get rid of people who are inappropriately obstructing a process that the organisation knows must happen, but in the NHS you normally have to keep them in post, and it may be years before their negative effect works its way out of the system. It has been said that corporate mergers take 10 years to settle down and have everybody working for the common goal. I suspect that is an underestimate. One of the added problems is that the NHS has no established arbitration process for resolving merger issues, the prelude to mergers can therefore become even more acrimonious than it might, with long-term ill effects.[2]

One might reasonably think the common goal is the care of patients. Sad to say the tribal reflexes of groups in the NHS seeking to preserve their identity, their traditions and their original territories will all too often overwhelm that basic principle. Lack of enthusiasm for mergers is not solely the province of doctors and patients as is sometimes claimed. A survey of 500 senior NHS managers by the Institute of Health Services Management found that "one out of every three managers believed that the drive for mergers was purely politically motivated and 93% believed them to be disruptive, 73% disagreed with NHS research that claimed that hospitals with less than 300 beds are uneconomic." Hardly the responses one would hope to see in the group central to the implementation of mergers but this is not surprising. Doctors and nurses rarely lose their jobs during mergers, managers do and even if they do not they may have to weather an uncomfortable period when there is uncertainty about their future, they may have to apply for their own jobs in the new joint organisation. It is hardly surprising therefore that unless the futures of at least the senior management team are settled right at the beginning of a merger process, the very people who need to make it happen will be less than fully committed to the task.

All in all it must be best to avoid mergers if possible, as they can fuel instability and anxiety and rarely achieve their objectives. "It is not at all clear from the evidence whether such marriages are "made in heaven" or are simply politically convenient as a perceived "quick fix" which ultimately deflects attention from difficult choices about Health Care priorities".[3] Even citing quality gain as a justification for mergers is difficult to substantiate from published evidence. In the USA where efficiency gains are cited as evidence that a merger is necessary some proposed mergers have been challenged in court which usually found the cases unpersuasive on the evidence offered.

There are some basic principles which could help mergers work, but they seem only rarely to be applied:

- Do very, very careful research to determine whether merger is necessary.
- Involve all the key players early.
- Define the plan and stick to it.
- Make senior appointments to the new merged unit early and with a minimum duration of uncertainty.
- Communicate, communicate, communicate.
- FUND IT!

6.3 RATIONING

Rationing of healthcare of course exists, it always did and always will. The problem with rationing in the NHS is that the current systems for rationing are "inefficient, inequitable, undemocratic and opaque".[4] Anyone who works within the Health Service knows this to be the case and knows how subtle rationing can be. For example, the old lady who does not call her GP because she considers him to be too busy. The GP who does not refer her to hospital with her renal failure because he believes that limited resources should not be used to dialyse old ladies in renal failure; the unwillingness to order a test for her because the waiting list for such tests is too long. The inability for her to see a nephrologist because nephrologists are in such short supply and so on. We have all lived with this state of affairs for many years, but doctors, managers and particularly doctor/managers, become more frustrated by it as the pressures to ration increase and an increasing openness in society makes it inescapable that one must admit that it is happening and explain why. This state of affairs is made worse by consecutive governments none of whom has had the courage to admit the reality of the situation, who have twisted and turned and talked as

203

if the managerial revolution or efficiency or prioritisation or mergers or the private finance initiative, or even when all that fails, a little more cash will solve the problem. In 1994, Duncan Nichol who had been Chief Executive of the NHS and presumably could have been expected to understand how the NHS worked, established a group to stimulate debate about the future of the NHS and rationing and to clarify policy. That group concluded, not unreasonably, that rationing would be necessary. Yet Stephen Dorrell, the Secretary of State at that time, inappropriately quoting H.L. Mencken, said Nichol's group's analysis was "simple, obvious and wrong".

Demand for healthcare and new options for providing healthcare expand faster than provision and, whatever government ministers may say, sooner or later explicit rationing will have to come into play. I have a thick file crammed with papers and comment saying just this. Some date back many years yet none of them announces a realistic government-driven initiative to explore a common national framework in which limited health resources can be used efficiently and equitably. The British habit of "muddling through" appears to be the officially sanctioned policy.

This does not mean there is not action, and indeed some of the actions are driven by central government, but they are few and none of the actions have led to a structure whereby clinical managers have a consistent set of administrative rules by which they respond to inadequate provision. That responsibility has been devolved to separate health authorities and to a plethora of different sticking plaster remedies, the only point of this process being that the health authority outside the hospital and managers inside the hospital are demonised as the agents of rationing. Since there is no central acknowledgement of the need to ration, any rationing that actually occurs is perceived as a fault of the hospital, a dereliction of duty by the manager or bloody-mindedness by the doctor. There is no immediate end to this in sight, so to help the medical manager understand why she will remain in the mire, the remainder of this section deals with current means by which resource use is restrained and then a discussion on some of the areas which the medical manager's successors will need to watch in the future.

6.3.1 Current mechanisms of rationing

The primary agent in rationing is the fixed budget. This in subtle or unsubtle format works from the top of the NHS to the bottom.

The rationing of surgical care by waiting list is perhaps the clearest example; the inability to afford beds and operating time leads to a waiting list. It does indeed force an increase in day surgery and shorter stays but these do not suffice and the waiting list remains in place. Health authorities could earmark more money to reduce the waiting list if they judged the operations present on the waiting list to be of sufficient clinical importance and the regular panic event of the "waiting list initiative" shows what can be achieved, but in most prioritisation exercises the treatment of low urgency surgical problems does not score highly. Health purchasing authorities may simply ration by allocating an inadequate global budget, but in most instances they now attempt to be more pro-active and specify how their finite budget is to be used by providers of care. They may put a ceiling on the number of interventions or the type of interventions which are allowed. In making that sort of judgment the issues are normally considered extremely carefully in a multidisciplinary debate informed by judgments about efficacy and importance and the needs of the specific population that the purchaser serves. But however carefully the exercise is carried out there will always be patients left outside; that is what rationing is about. You can fudge the issue by not being too explicit and by not insisting that a decision should cover everyone in the population but all that does is push the decision-making process back to where it always was with the clinician. In the meantime, all that has happened is that excluded patients get angry. This can happen even in apparently non-contentious decisions. Lewisham, Southwark and Lambeth Health Authority has been threatened with judicial review by HIV organisations after removing complementary medicine and osteopathy from a list of interventions it will purchase. Explicit decisions tend to be at the margins, as Klein observes: "the price of visibility is triviality".[5] Even so lack of central support for the principle of exclusion means that even where you have a policy that excludes the excision of sebaceous cysts and tattoos, the doctor is left having to argue the toss with the patient or the manager to argue the toss with the clinician. If the sebaceous cyst not worthy of operation turns out to be a bizarre and atypical sarcoma, then God help you; the lawyers and the NHS Executive won't.

Many health authorities recently looked very carefully at whether they could and should fund the use of beta interferon for the treatment of multiple sclerosis. For most regions in the country the cost of this was expected to run into millions of pounds a year and many health authorities decided that this was not an appropriate use of funds; there might be some benefit from the treatment but it was going to be small in relation to the amount of money that the treatment would cost. This decision was made usually by a mix of managers and clinicians, and to be frank was not a difficult decision to make, either scientifically or in public health terms. In a managerial sense the health authorities were simply doing what the Government had asked them to do, take local decisions about the use of resources. North Derbyshire Health Authority were taken to Court by a patient to whom this funding was denied, citing a government circular which indicated there were circumstances in which some patients should have the drug provided. The health authority lost the case and the whole principle of devolved decision making about rationing became to some extent a nonsense.

The much reported case of Jamie B is another example of attempts at rationing by an individual health authority being unsupported. Cambridgeshire and Huntingdon Health Authority made what they believed to be a good moral and clinical case for not funding yet more chemotherapy for this child with terminal leukaemia, but the patient's relatives and the media thought otherwise and the unfortunate and unsupported health authority became victims of the lack of clarity about how rationing decisions should be made. The Chief Executive's reflections on the case make instructive reading. His conclusions reflecting on the experience were that:

> Making decisions on issues of such profound importance to citizens, is a matter for government, indeed a matter for national debate and resolution.

> The quality of the process by which decisions are arrived at is as important as the actual outcomes. The process requires explicit documentation of clinical evidence, self-confidence, compassion and a preparedness to communicate these widely.[6]

However it is always going to be difficult for a bureaucratic organisation, primarily perceived as dealing in cash rather than patients, to make difficult decisions. In theory, it may be easier for fundholding GPs, or their primary care successors to deny treatment. This nevertheless has the moral difficulty of putting the doctor in the invidious position of making financially based judgments about rationing which might be different from his clinical judgments. That is, nevertheless, what we have all been doing for many years. What is different now is that we are expected to be open about it and thus abused for it. This is the nub of the problem. Whatever the gymnastics that have preceded a decision to limit access to treatment, the final decision is properly and normally made by clinicians and is thus properly a repeated exercise in clinical judgment, not just an exercise in policing lists drawn up by health authorities. Nevertheless, whereas allocation decisions were made privately and quietly in good faith in the past, they can now only be sustained when made openly, honestly and in public if the individual clinician's decisions are set against a national rationing framework which has been properly debated and publicly accepted and which admits a need for doctors to make decisions about allocation.

So where does the medical manager go from here? Firstly she needs to keep an eye on the debate. At the moment, because the Government does not engage in it the debate is akin to Dutch Protestants planning the future of the Church of Rome, but perhaps things will change. Secondly, the debate as published is likely to be confusing, diffuse and circular to the average reader. I challenge anyone to get any sense of satisfaction or any perception of progress out of a review of the last 5 years' articles on rationing in the *British Medical Journal*![7]

6.3.2 The future of rationing—steps to watch

(a) A better decision-taking process
A better and agreed process for decision taking at local level will need to be established when central government does not take these decisions (the removal of dental services and eye tests, the closure of psychiatric institutions and the limiting of breast screening to women under 65 are, it should be remembered, central rationing decisions). Local processes will need to be very open, very well informed by an evidence base that looks not just at outcome in a life expectancy sense but also more at quality. Nevertheless on balance most opinion seems to support the necessity of central decision making about major rationing issues so as to avoid the "rationing by postcode" which occurs when different health authorities make different decisions. Thus the lady in one

street has access to Taxol to treat her advanced malignancy whereas the friend she made in hospital being treated for the same disease but living in a different health authority's jurisdiction does not.

(b) A more intelligent national debate

There is a need for a more intelligent national debate on what core services the NHS should supply. What mechanism should be used to decide what is in the core?[8] New Zealand, Norway, Oregon and Holland have all famously addressed these issues, none with satisfactory outcomes, and none in a similar way. Oregon established a prioritised list of treatments and have funded the best 565 of 696 options. Holland refined the process by which decisions would be made and identified effectiveness and efficiency as crucial limiters, but like everyone else simply ended up rationing services like homoeopathy and adult dental care (Figure 6.4). However both Holland and New Zealand rejected the excluding nature of the Oregon exercise and fixed on the establishment of guidelines for clinical care based on consensus conferences. The basic tenet is "only provide what works". All these exercises involved the public in the debate. The British Government seems to prefer to move in the direction of the New Zealand initiative with the stress on guidelines, hoping somehow to restrict treatment which a formal evaluation process does not find "clinically effective". It has even set up an organisation to make judgments about what is clinically effective. With chillingly Orwellian overtones the organisation will be acronymically NICE: the National Institute for Clinical Effectiveness. There are other groups in the UK looking objectively at the problem and these may promulgate usable alternative options. An example is the Rationing Agenda Group who have already published on the subject.[9]

(c) Involvement of the public

A lot of lip service is attached to the need to involve the public, but how to involve them in a meaningful rather than token way is more difficult. Focus groups are fashionable but of course undemocratic; conferences with lay participation similarly. It is however known that the public are prepared to display altruism and understand that some members may have to forego some care to allow the proper treatment of sicker others. Additionally, the public is known to be unhappy about local rather than national processes being used for rationing. Lastly the public does expect

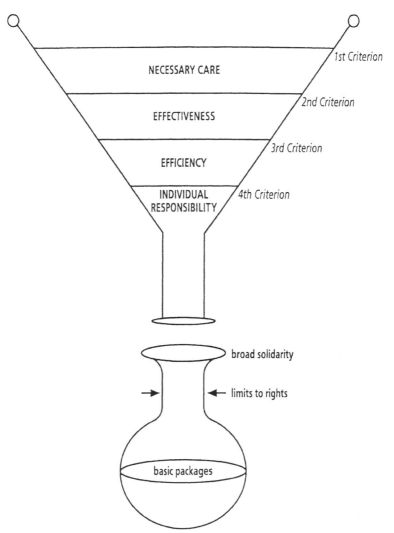

Figure 6.4 The conceptual framework proposed by the Dunning Committee to determine healthcare priorities. The much quoted "Dunning Filter" filtered out much the same avoidable care as others have proposed: adult dental care, homoeopathic medicine, etc.

to be involved.[10] When they are involved their priorities differ somewhat from those of GPs and of consultants, but not hugely.[11] The exact process by which the public can declare its preferences for healthcare might start from a proposal made by Ronald Dworkin, an American professor of law and a medical ethicist. Professor Dworkin proposed that the public should be asked to imagine a world with five characteristics:

(1) That everybody has the same amount of money to spend.
(2) That information about medicine and its effectiveness is accurate and freely available.
(3) That everybody's interests, children, adults and the elderly, are put at the same level.
(4) That everyone is assumed to be at the same risk of disease.
(5) That people make decisions rationally.

In this imaginary world people would need to buy an imaginary insurance policy but would have to specify what was to be covered by that policy. Professor Dworkin argued that for example few would buy a health insurance policy that offered them lifesaving treatment if they fell into a persistent vegetative state, nor did he think that there would be many takers for a policy that offered lifesaving treatment in the late stages of dementia and so on. A number of interventions currently regularly provided would quickly be excluded. His predictions may or may not be true but the idealistic scenario which he presents illustrates an academically reasonable starting point for a debate.[12] If the public is to be involved the media will play a large part in influencing its views. At the moment the media is so immature and sensationalist in its attitude to the health issue that it could be dangerously counter-productive to involve it.

Realistically, public debate may do a little to control demand and will not increase supply unless it acquiesces to tax increases but it might help increase the acceptability of gaps between supply and demand and the practical mechanics of administering rationing. The sceptic will nevertheless point out that the public as a healthy generality, and the patient as a sick specific, differ widely in their opinions. The public as a whole is very likely to say that the millions earmarked for the use of beta interferon for a remitting disease might be better spent elsewhere. The MS Society and the patient with an acute exacerbation of his MS might disagree. What this points to is the problem of who shall be the responsible agent for taking the recommendations of NICE or of citizen's juries and enforcing them in the clinic?

(d) A radical rethink about how the NHS delivers care

This seems the unlikely horse at the back of the field carrying too heavy an ideological burden to give it a chance of winning, but you never know. If it does put in a showing perhaps it will be along the lines of the NHS contracting to provide only truly core services and requiring individuals to insure themselves if they want the remainder. Weale pointed out that in a world of limited resources we have to resolve an *inconsistent triad*, "a collection of propositions any two of which are compatible with each other but which when viewed together in a threesome form a contradiction".[13] He implies that we can have one of the three possible pairs in the triad of comprehensiveness, quality and availability. We can have either:

- A comprehensive service of high quality but not available to all (as in the USA).

or

- A comprehensive service freely available to all but not of high quality (the NHS).

or

- A high-quality service freely available to all but not comprehensive (i.e. excellent core coverage but no more).

(e) New technology assessment

Technology is the military arm of science, it articulates our preference for action over inaction and adsorbs our obsession with the new. It is also expensive and often harmful. Even if the current allocation for healthcare were sufficient and there was no rationing, one could be fairly certain that the advent of new technologies and new drugs, new high-cost procedures, or new low-cost high-volume procedures would upset the applecart in the future. The problem at the moment is that these new arrivals can take root at hospital level with minimal control, usually without a formal business plan or consultation with purchasers, even without consultation with other groups within the hospital such as a prescribing committee, a clinical director or the director of finance who might have a view. The new technology simply insinuates itself and provides a constant pressure on resources. If we were able to control these new technologies and use the ones which were truly valuable, and

211

were able to make a judgment about them *before* they began to be implemented widely in hospitals we might have a humane rationing weapon. The beta interferon story might never have arisen. There are many examples of widespread inappropriate and expensive use of new technology before its assessment. For example laparoscopic repair of inguinal hernias. Inguinal hernias can of course normally be repaired as a day-case under local anaesthetic with minimal discomfort and an early return to work. Laparoscopic hernia repairs require a general anaesthetic, an invasion of the abdominal cavity, the use of disposable instruments whose cost exceeds the current total cost of an outpatient hernia operation; and all this to produce an operation whose only benefit in a first-time unilateral hernia is possibly to return the patients to work a day or so earlier, though that is unproven. The drive for its use is clinicians looking for novelty (kindly called innovators), pressure from instrument companies, clinicians wishing not to be left behind and sometimes possibly hospitals wishing to show that they are doing "up-to-date" things. If new technology assessment as a form of rationing is to take root, then much more mature media reporting is going to be needed. At present the media are perfectly prepared to report enthusiastically on totally spurious, unvalidated alternative therapies for cancer, etc., so one wonders how they might respond to limitation of a slightly effective but very expensive treatment which is to be withheld.

(f) Demand management

This is as much to do with education and access to information as anything. The use of telephone helplines for example can be shown to reduce call outs of doctors and attendances at accident and emergency departments. Better education might reduce the expectation that to be effective the GP needs to prescribe something or to refer to a hospital.[14]

(g) The practicalities

Much of what is written on rationing is academic and fixes on the "what" not the "how". For the foreseeable future the medical manager will be the bouncer at the door as far as rationing is concerned. There is no prospect of this task becoming any easier so what advice can the medical manager be given?

212

- If there are explicit restrictions make sure they are in writing and that you know who they came from and the process by which they were established.
- Make sure that restrictions do not include a blanket exclusion unless it is for good evidence-based reasons which you can support.
- Try to obtain or provide written information that can be given to patients explaining the reasons behind the decision.
- Ensure equitable access to any reduced service. This was predominantly a problem in relation to GP fundholders but will persist for as long as different health authorities make different rationing decisions.
- Try to limit rationing to procedures not groups of people, i.e. avoid hard boundaries which can always be argued as illogical but allow space for evidence-based medicine to have a role if its findings are explicit. For example the denial of certain vascular surgical interventions to smokers, not because these smokers are smokers, but because the procedures will not work if they continue to smoke.
- Argue for services based on respect for humanity, not just simple life expectancy, even though this brings you back into the difficult area of "gender reassignment", infertility treatment, and mastopexy.
- Carry the clinicians with you.
- Always be prepared to revisit the decision.

6.4 IT/COMPUTERS

The Health Service is not a supermarket and is not an airline. When it comes to information technology (IT) this is unfortunate! IT ought to be central to the smooth running of the Health Service where 20–30% of employees' time is spent processing information, i.e. where at any one time 250 000 people are handling data. Supermarkets and airlines, though less important to society than the Health Service, are threaded through with sophisticated computer systems without which they would function less effectively or not at all. The Health Service should be in their league but by any measure you care to take it is not only not winning it is not even playing. The NHS spends £250 million on IT each year which at less than 0.1% of turnover is substantially less than the 2% of turnover that commercial organisations expect to spend. The Audit

213

Commission looked at the use of IT in 15 NHS hospitals in 1995 and found to no one's surprise that it was unsatisfactory. They did however produce a useful analysis of the failure, pointing out among other problems the lack of clinical leadership.[15]

As a doctor and particularly as a doctor/manager you will daily be frustrated by the incompatibility and inadequacies of the computer systems you will have to rely on; their age, their lack of sophistication, their slow unsympathetic formats. Rather than just complain and walk away you ought to do your bit to try and make it better, because it is doctors and doctors in management who I would submit are partly to blame for the present unhappy situation.

6.4.1 The underlying problem

Outsiders say that the Health Service's computer problem is fourfold. It is inadequately capitalised, there is a lack of clarity about what is needed, a lack of central authority to guide development and a lack of good staff to implement it. Something that is politely summarised as "an immature business environment".

The arguments about the central control of computing development can in fairness be played either way, for or against. It is easy to construe as a stupendous failure the fact that the NHS did not see years ago the need to develop a set of software to match the basic needs that are common to all hospitals. Software which would allow one hospital and organisation to talk to another using the same data sets, the same security arrangements, etc. What one may assume to have been simply financial or planning cowardice could equally, however, be viewed historically as prudence, for what sallies into central planning there have been tended to have unhappy outcomes if the blind and malodorous alley of the Read code debacle is anything to go by.

6.4.2 IT in your hospital

Most hospitals have an IT department; either a man and his techno-dog or a bigger one with grander but more opaque titles like "deputy systems engineer" (no it's not my job to fix your PC) and "corporate network planner" (no you can't connect your PC to the Internet). What many lack is a clear purpose.

214

The clear IT purpose (or lack of)

If your hospital's IT strategy is clear and workable and works, well done! (can I have a second opinion, please doctor?), but *don't* skip to the next chapter, things can still go wrong. If your hospital's IT strategy is, heaven forbid, less than clear, then as like or not you will find it has been jointly drafted by a senior computer nerd, the director of finance and a doctor brought in "because he knows about computers" (i.e. has an Apple Mac at home). What should perhaps have happened is something like this:

Stage One: Strategy should be set based purely on management and clinical criteria. No computer input is needed at this stage and I would beg to suggest that there is an advantage at this stage of excluding anybody with an interest in or knowledge of computers. Only when the needs have been defined as a brief prioritised list should the computer people be set loose on it.

Stage Two: Now it gets more difficult because having defined the outline requirements of what you want you will need, in consultation with the computer people, to decide for each problem:

(1)   Whether it *can* be computerised.
(2)   Whether it *needs* to be computerised.
(3)   Whether it needs to link with other systems.
(4)   Where in the sequence of developments it will be placed.

There are separate strands here which need to be interwoven as the process evolves. A computer person will need to ensure that a system can be achieved within the defined cost and is technically feasible and a clinician/manager/nurse, etc. will need to define the exact user specification. In this last context in my experience it has been very difficult to recruit doctors to spend the considerable time and energy on system development that is needed at the specification stage, and if you do recruit someone it is often difficult to get them to fix on what is practical and achievable. The detailed "Statement of Need" produced for a new test ordering and reporting system for our trust ran to 87 pages. That sort of effort requires real time and commitment from clinicians.

Most hospital trusts need computing for ten core activities.

(1) Payroll.
(2) Personnel.
(3) Patients master index.

215

(4) Finance.
(5) Scheduling of theatres, clinics, X-rays, etc.
(6) Ordering tests and seeing the results.
(7) Waiting list management.
(8) Bed management.
(9) Core information (clinical protocols, drug data, etc.).
(10) Communication.

These are all products, i.e. they require an end point. You will find that many of your colleagues are keen to record all sorts of audit and activity data on computer and may need to be reminded that high-volume ephemeral data in general costs more to enter than is justified and it is rarely retrieved.

There is an enormous amount of data sloshing around in any healthcare system. The Audit Commission estimates that about a quarter of doctors' and nurses' time is spent collecting data and using it.[16] What part of this would be better managed with the use of computer systems is unknown. Enthusiasts will say that it is self-evident that computers must be used for all these tasks but Lock, in a review of the published literature,[17] found only scanty objective evidence to support that view. He concluded that certain benefits are however likely to accrue from the use of computers and cited:

- Easier access to the medical history and the results of tests.
- Easier and quicker generation of letters and discharge summaries.
- Support for protocols and guidelines.
- Support for shared care between professionals.

Some current and expensive developments such as PACS (picture archiving and communication system) which seem to be just to do with imaging systems are in reality just another IT project needing all the planning, wide consultation and adequate initial investment that other IT systems demand.[18]

The role of the clinician/manager
Clinicians involved in planning systems need to use their clinical knowledge and experience to judge what information *needs* to be processed and bear in mind that ideally data should be recorded at the moment that it happens and the recording should be a normal part of clinical/managerial care. In the Health Service which has traditionally been labour intensive we have a fixation on

216

manually entered data: bar codes rarely get a look in. I'm not saying all patients should have bar codes tattooed on their bottoms, but supermarkets handle huge volumes of data infinitely better than we do and the bar code is inseparable from that. We're told as usual that the capital cost prohibits progress.

The clinician in management needs to do his bit to ensure that things go well in planning computer systems. I would submit that the medical manager has a responsibility to be very hard-nosed both with the IT department and more particularly with his colleagues when it comes to planning systems. Here are some questions that you might ask:

(1) Do we really need this system?
(2) Will it really save money? (This is not an absolute requirement but it helps to obtain the funding.)

You should be aware of the "boys with toys" phenomenon in computer systems. Clinicians are just as prone to this disease as non-clinicians, possibly more so. The "boys with toys" phenomenon occurs where an individual or group decide they need a computer system because it seems interesting, exciting, up-to-date, fashionable—"sexy". Their enthusiasm may outrun managerial pragmatism. The infant always "*needs*" the thing it *wants* mummy. In trying to understand whether the need is real one may be frustrated by an unholy alliance in this between the doctor who wants the new toy and the computer people inside who want a sexy project and the supplier outside who wants the contract signed and who will promise the earth to get it. Remember what happened to Dr Faust and be very hard-nosed! You the manager are more dependent on computer outputs than other clinicians. You can only make effective decisions if you have accurate aggregated clinical data, so you need to ensure that systems are robust.

Here are some more hard-nosed questions to ask:

(1) Given the limited availability of finance do you want this system in preference to some other expenditure which is not computer related?
(2) Do the systems which you already have and which are central to your business actually work properly or would the money be better spent on improving them?
(3) Does the system you are proposing require planned replacement? If so how will you fund it?

217

(4) Will you be able to afford the support costs?

(5) Do you need staff specifically to run the system?

Sad to say my experience is that however hard you try your organisation will buy at least one system that it cannot afford, does not need and which does not work. You *will* be a victim!

You will be a victim

Most clinicians don't understand computer technology in any real way nor appreciate the speed of its change, nor have an in-depth understanding of what is achievable, so it is easy to take us for a ride. At the very least during that ride which may, of course, be exciting we should ask our helmeted, wild-eyed, Mr Toad who is driving about:

(1) Software documentation—will it be unavailable or available but incomprehensible as usual?

(2) Support—will it be adequate? Whizz kids whizz off elsewhere, software firms go bust or get taken over.

(3) May we assume that the system you are implementing will always work more slowly than you want and security will be non-existent because Nurse Blogg's access code has been written in indelible ink beside the computer screen so that all the agency nurses can use it?

(4) When the system needs to be expanded because the original specification was poorly written will there be enough digits in the codes, enough free hand space in the forms, and generally enough leeway in the software and the hardware?

(5) Have you clearly identified the suppliers' liabilities if the system doesn't work as they claim? Have the suppliers tried contractually to limit their liabilities and have we taken steps to protect ourselves against that?

When eventually Mr Toad gets you to his destination and you emerge shaken and poorer but with a spanking new computer system make sure you have arranged to have an objective review in 6 months' or a year's time, and if it really is not good enough, appropriate enough, flexible enough and is costing you more and more in support and modification have the perspicacity to junk it there and then.

I must apologise to the reader for this section having been couched in such negative terms, but as most of what you will read elsewhere about computers and computing in the Health Service tends to skirt around the snags, no apology is really needed. One hopes new developments will be of proportionately more value for patient care, for example telemedicine, the medical uses of the Internet, and the NHS network itself. There are lots of genuinely useful and exciting developments in computing within the Health Service and the single message I would want to finish with is that doctors and doctor managers have a critical role in ensuring that these developments are appropriate and workable, so do not be put off by what I have said above, just be wary.

6.5 RISK AND RISK MANAGEMENT

We live in an age of fear; not real fear of death and starvation, penury and war but a corrosive anxiety that in any situation the worst will happen, that nothing is safe and no one and no thing or principle is to be trusted.[19] The environment that this insecurity spawns generates numberless attempts to regulate and check what has happened or what might happen and convoluted attempts to minimise any risk that an individual or organisation might fall prey to. You could say this habit is simply wise caution or you could see it as a loss of trust and self confidence. Whatever your interpretation it is for now a fact of life that one must manage risk actively and centrally. Between 1967 and 1972, "risk" was cited about 1000 times in medical journals; between 1992 and 1997 "risk" has been cited 80 000 times. There are now journals, specialist lawyers, management advisers and conference organisers all living off the phenomenon of "risk". As a doctor the major risks that will concern you are the risks to patients flowing from inept clinical care. A person in hospital faces a 1 in 200 risk of significant error compared with a 1 in 2 000 000 risk on an aeroplane.[20] There are also "Health and Safety" issues relating to the general hospital environment, the handling of toxic chemicals, waste disposal, fire escapes, etc., etc., etc. Hospitals were once under "Crown Immunity" which allowed them to take a cavalier approach to Health and Safety issues, but that immunity has gone; Health and Safety inspectors now visit hospitals although since 1988 there have been only 40 successful prosecutions for breaches of hygiene and for unsafe equipment. This small number probably simply reflects a softly softly approach by the Health and Safety Inspectorate. The pace is hotting up and in 1997 the Chief

Executive of the Swindon and Marlborough Trust resigned after the trust was found guilty of a breach of Health and Safety regulations. It is a salutary lesson about hospitals' relationships with the National Audit Office that that Trust was one of those voluntarily participating in a study of accidents in hospital by the National Audit Office. District auditors looked at accidents in 30 NHS acute trusts during May and June 1995.[21] They discovered that more than half the trusts did not have incident recording systems, but even so they felt able to calculate that there were about half a million accidents each year in acute hospital trusts in England and Wales. Three-quarters of the accidents involved patients and visitors and 80% were due to slips, trips and falls. Among the staff most of the recorded accidents were needlestick injuries (of which of course only a minute fraction are reported). Nurses take 360 000 days' sick leave per year for reasons of occupational health or injury. Only half of trusts comply with more than 70% of legislation on health and safety. Most of this is not your business as a clinical manager but the need to reduce *clinical* risk most emphatically is.

All hospitals need a *programme of risk management*. This does not mean bussing in expensive risk management consultants to tell you what you know or can find out for yourself but cannot afford to put right. Fundamentally it means a drive to change the culture away from passive risk acceptance to active risk prevention.

"Risk management" sounds commercial even slightly disreputable, as if you cared about the risk to the organisation rather than the victim. Doctors are almost unwittingly involved in a continuous process of risk management all the time though on a small scale. Do I need to get a haemoglobin? Do all patients over 50 need a preoperative chest X-ray? Can I discount the possibility that this patient will have a side effect from the drug I am about to prescribe? What are the risks of not admitting this patient now but waiting until tomorrow? Risk management is simply that activity generalised onto the whole organisation's business. The phrase "risk management" is a good one because it accepts that risks cannot be obviated and that the organisation must admit the ever-present sword of Damocles but try to arrange its business to minimise the risk of it falling and minimise the damage when it does.

A considered review of most hospitals' risk environment would probably show that the string holding Damocles' sword has been sawn nine-tenths through and the bulk of the hospital staff and patients marshalled into a huddle directly beneath it. Hospitals are dangerous places, they are full of malevolent bacteria, surgeons, unrestrained technology, radiation, partly trained agency nurses, junior doctors half asleep and equipment that is years beyond its date for replacement. Yet we affect not to notice. The real risk is that risk management is seen merely as another chore which will cost us money, upset people and take up valuable time that could be better spent doing something else. The slightly pernickety, nannyish attitude of the bureaucrats who administer "Health and Safety" issues and their frequent inability to understand the hierarchy of risks in a hospital makes this the agenda item greeted with a groan.

Your organisation may have faced up to these issues, but if not a way forward might include the following:

(1) Change the mind set of employees so that they see risks and faults not as the responsibility of reprehensible individuals but as an institutional issue requiring institutional solutions. Also change the attitude to error so as to see adverse events as valuable indicators of how the organisation functions at its core as well as at its tatty edges.

(2) Establish a risk management committee. Yes I know it is another committee and we don't want extra committees but this is an exception. It should have on it at least the chief executive, the director of nursing and the medical director and should report either to the board or the executive. It may be appropriate to establish as a subcommittee a group of clinicians looking specifically at issues of *clinical* risk.

(3) Examine all the areas of the institution's business (with help from outside consultants if you must) and identify high-risk areas. Prioritise them for action.

(4) Set an action plan and explicitly require clinicians and managers to attend to the identified problems within a specified timescale.

(5) Raise the general awareness of risk in the organisation by involving as many staff as possible in the process of risk assessment and management and by publishing your findings, actions and outcomes.

(6) Have a formal procedure available whereby staff may notify risks that they encounter (Figure 6.5).

221

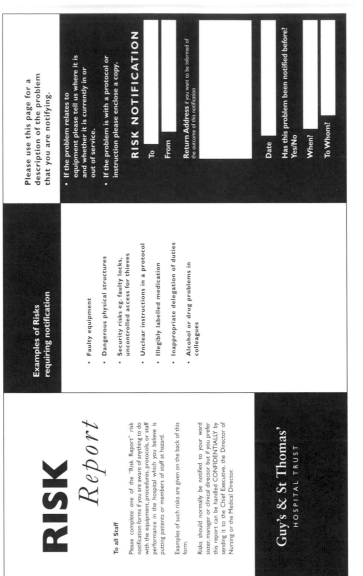

Figure 6.5 All hospitals need to encourage their staff to identify risk and to deal with it or notify it using a simple form such as this.

(7) Ensure that the director of finance understands that risk to patients equates to financial risk to the organisation, and persuade him that money spent on risk management is likely to save him money spent on litigation later.

6.5.1 High-risk areas

Many of the breaches of health and safety regulations or accidents are trivial or are not the result of any negligence by the trust. By contrast there are some high-risk areas and correcting these may require money, sometimes a lot of money; and there is no separately identified funding for this. Trust managers have the unenviable task of assessing the severity of risk and then balancing the need for expenditure to reduce low-level risks to staff, patients and visitors against more predictable benefits from spending the money on high-grade risks or on direct patient care. We are not allowed publicly to admit the frustrations of being told by health and safety people that such and such a risk which we perceive as trivial, *must* be immediately dealt with; yet there is no finance to cover the cost. To inform them in the execution of this balancing act all trusts need explicit "risk management" arrangements and an awareness of the magnitude of the different risks in human terms.

Common sense, clinical knowledge, a review of litigation claims and of complaints, together with a reading of back-numbers of the *Risk Management Journal*, will identify some common threads that run through the highest areas of real risk in most hospitals and other health institutions (Figure 6.6). Insofar as the clinical care of patients is concerned high-risk areas are:

(1) Obstetrics and orthopaedics. In these there is a crucial need for agreed and adhered to protocols and close supervision of junior doctors.[22]
(2) Locums and their induction, agency nurses.
(3) Inadequate note keeping and storage of records.
(4) Uncorrected faults in equipment.
(5) Inadequate hand-over from doctor to doctor and nurse to nurse at shift change.
(6) Activities outside the normal area for the institution.
(7) Inappropriate delegation and working beyond personal competence levels.
(8) Drug mistakes.
(9) Failure to act on the results of pathology and imaging tests.

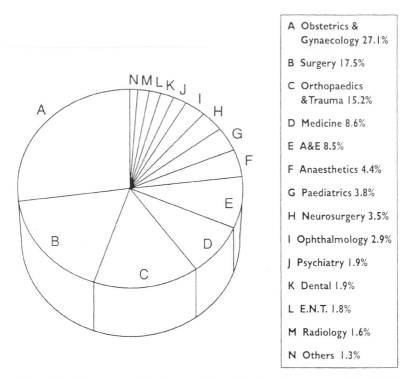

A Obstetrics &
   Gynaecology 27.1%

B Surgery 17.5%

C Orthopaedics
   &Trauma 15.2%

D Medicine 8.6%

E A&E 8.5%

F Anaesthetics 4.4%

G Paediatrics 3.8%

H Neurosurgery 3.5%

I Ophthalmology 2.9%

J Psychiatry 1.9%

K Dental 1.9%

L E.N.T. 1.8%

M Radiology 1.6%

N Others 1.3%

Figure 6.6   The spectrum of negligence claims. This chart shows an analysis of 1000 claims made over a 5-year period (1990–95) and analysed by Dr Armond Gwynne for the solicitors Bevan Ashford. The claims are divided up by percentage per specialty. Obstetrics and gynaecology have the most instances and these are also the most expensive to settle.

Not all of these risks are, of course, truly within your province as a medical manager, but there are some areas where doctors need to take the lead, particularly in specifying who can be safely allowed to do what, for example how to flatten the nasty bit of the learning curve in endoscopic surgery. Some areas of risk may require you the clinical manager, now or in the future, to take some difficult decisions which are difficult to implement and which may widen the gulf between you and your clinical colleagues. The issue of certification and deciding who shall and shall not be allowed to undertake procedures within a hospital is the most contentious in this area, the most visible aspect of which is the surgeon who performs a wide range of operations some of them only infrequently. We know from published data that, for example, there is a substantial excess mortality from undertaking only a small number of oesophagectomies or pancreatectomies a year. Most surgeons recognise this difficulty but it is difficult to stop and all sorts of specious arguments will be put to you, claiming for example that a particular individual's performance is better than average so she's safe or that she needs to retain a breadth of experience so that she can be on-call. A more difficult area involves the undertaking of new or innovative procedures where unwillingness to take a risk will hamper progress.

We and lawyers tend to think of risk as being inherent in specifics, people, equipment or protocols, but we need to remember that there are features of the organisation itself which are recognised as increasing risk; in particular rapid change, poor morale, inadequate communications, and a high workload.[23]

The risks inherent in doctors' incompetence or illness are dealt with in Sections 4.6 to 4.8.

6.5.2 The costs of neglecting risk

Although only 0.5% of the NHS budget is spent on risk management, a successful claim against your trust can have potentially dramatic implications for its finances. It is not uncommon for obstetric claims to exceed £1 million. Of this the fraction representing 0.5% of the trust's annual revenue must be paid by the trust, the remainder must be borrowed from the Treasury and repaid with interest within 10 years. The NHS LA (NHS Litigation Authority) will negotiate structured settlements in these cases. NHS trusts are forbidden from taking out commercial insurance to protect themselves against these kind of risks but there exists the Clinical Negligence Scheme for Trusts (CNST) which is a cooperative system within the Health Service which helps to spread the risks. Not everyone has joined this and it quite properly has some stringent entrance requirements requiring risk management procedures to be in place.

6.5.3 The future

Risk and error are not phenomena about to be "solved". The Harvard Medical Practice Study found 3.7% of admissions involved an adverse event, and in 1% of admissions care was judged to be negligent and to have contributed to permanent disability or the death of the patient.[24] That is probably a very low figure, an Australian study found that 16.6% of admissions resulted in an adverse event.[25] Another study proposed that there are 100 000 deaths per year in the USA from adverse drug reactions, a suspiciously round figure![26] Currently, only a tiny proportion of these are documented or acted upon. Even so it is claimed that it would cost as much as £1 billion to settle the UK's outstanding negligence cases.[27]

6.6 EDUCATION VERSUS SERVICE

You would perhaps not expect to find a section on education in a book about clinicians and management. Most such books ignore it, yet experience as a medical manager shows that the impact of education on service and vice-versa is an everyday and difficult problem. Indeed the clinician in management may be on either side in the service versus education tussles, or indeed both, although rarely synchronously. For me the reality of the potential clashes was evident from the day when I became clinical director of surgery and was politely asked by my colleagues to give up the post of surgical tutor as the two posts were thought to have incompatible agendas.

Education versus service problems come up in two distinct area:

(1) The education of trainees.
(2) Undergraduate training.

The most difficult of these is the first.

6.6.1 Service commitments of trainees

Trainee doctors train predominantly on the job and for generations service as apprenticeship was the norm, and in most instances was the best. Many clinicians, possibly most clinicians, still believe this model to be the best; nevertheless the apprenticeship model which has lasted us well for many centuries is now under relentless pressure from reduced hours of work, from a faster turnover of patients, from a more "efficient" service which does not allow sufficient time for consultant and trainee to be together and lastly, in many instances, from the trend to a "consultant-based" as distinct from a "consultant-led" service. It sometimes seems there is also a confounding problem in that educationalists may seem not to perceive any virtue at all in the apprenticeship system. We have then, on the one hand, a host of clinicians and indeed many trainees, especially surgical ones, who believe that simply getting on with the job and being supervised for a proportion of the time is the way to learn. Set against, on the other hand, educationalists who believe that all trainees should be surplus to service requirements, that training should be predominantly formal and structured, and that a good deal of it should be gleaned away from the bedside. One has to be careful not to paint a picture of a battlefield that does not really exist, but these polarities are real so let us just say that the polarities lead to competing priorities for the medical manager who is once again pig in the middle and needs to address the conflicts.

The champions of educational priorities are the regional postgraduate deans, hospital postgraduate deans, universities, royal and other colleges and the various visiting teams that they all spawn. The rules of best educational practice to which these teams work are an amalgam of educational theory, educational fashion, government directives and financial rules to do with the holding of trainees' salaries. All of these are complicated and require special knowledge. These byways of the regulations to do with trainees are often bizarre, consisting of little known tracks between the NHS, universities, colleges, and medical schools. Special knowledge of this terrain breeds its own maquisards—small groups of activists determined to stand up for education against the crushing forces of finance driven service provision. They operate in small bands as visiting recognition teams, New Deal task forces, etc. Pitched battles are rare, victories small but progressive. Behind many of them is the shadowy but inspirational figure of Le Patron, the regional postgraduate dean. He is important because he controls the weaponry, the money that pays for these trainees and the recognition processes that allow hospitals to employ them. What are managers to do? The in-house finance people want efficiency savings and the purchasers want higher quality for lower cost 'and a consultant-based service. The colleges want more experience for trainees but the New Deal team wants them to work less hours. The university house officer inspection team wants the world to revolve around the house officer and newly empowered nurses want to take over the house officer's work. The whole jumble of competing requirements revolves on an endless merry-go-round. Every once in a while one of the teams comes to visit; you smile and wave and another comes by and you smile and wave until they've gone, because, in most instances, unfortunately you simply cannot square the circle. What each group wants is not compatible with what the other wants, so you smile and wave as they go by knowing that it will be at least a year before they are back and that most of their threats of withdrawal of recognition etc. simply aren't implementable because everyone else has the same problem. This is a sadly cynical attitude to take but it has for a long time been an unhappy state of affairs although it is slowly improving. The regional postgraduate deaneries are trying to ensure that incompatible demands are not made by different visiting teams, but unfortunately purchasers of healthcare (and that includes the Department of Health at origin) do not have mechanisms in place to ensure that adequate and funded time is set apart for both trainees and consultants to engage in formal educational processes. What they have done by contrast is insist that education occurs during the working week. The European Working Hours Directive will in time probably reduce this to 48 hours, which will add yet another dimension of difficulty to the problem.

The solutions to all this will, in the predictable future, have to remain compromises. The point at which service yields to education and vice-versa will no doubt move in a pendulum fashion. In the meantime the best the medical manager can do about it is not to see it as a battle, to remain on good terms with the educational teams and when involved in business planning he will need to do his best to write in the time and costs of education and keep education on the agenda, not only with the managerial side of the organisation but also with the clinicians.

That is very bland and will probably be insufficient in some areas where there will indeed be a battle between service and education which may resolve itself in two ways. The one most often threatened is that clinicians who do not teach and organisations who do not educate will lose their right to have trainees. Indeed it is possible that whole hospitals may in future be manned by consultants and "non-career grade" staff. For the educationalists there is of course also a risk in brinkmanship in that hospitals may say, as mine once had to about house surgeons in the New Deal, that the difficulties produced by the requirement to train and meet the hours requirements were so great that it was no longer in the organisation's interests to continue to offer that training. Many junior doctor tasks are now satisfactorily undertaken by nurses, and if their role is looked at completely cold-bloodedly, without any sympathy to the overall educational needs of the service, then they might indeed be considered expendable. The bluff worked.

At the other end of training there are anxieties for medical managers that the graduates from a Calman process which has not been developed enough to afford proper education will not be sufficiently trained to take on consultant posts. This is far from a theoretical worry and posts are already remaining unfilled, not through lack of applicants but through lack of properly trained applicants. Many of the trainees realise that this is a risk but are caught by the guillotine of European legislation which does not enable training to continue beyond what they decree appropriate. Our own trust wished to establish limited tenure post-Calman clinical fellowships; these have been extremely successful but against a background of vigorous rejection by the BMA worried about sub-consultant grades and enthusiasts for the Calman process who do not wish its wholeness to be undermined.

One is always wary of identifying more resources as the solution to problems, but most people conclude that the only solution to the current educational difficulties is to have sufficient extra staff available at consultant level to enable more formal educational time with trainees. There will in addition need to be structured education for trainers. Doctors are not professional teachers and they need to be taught to teach and to assess. Until that happy day the medical manager will have to continue to orchestrate the compromises.

6.6.2 Undergraduate teaching

The medical manager cannot become distanced from issues of undergraduate teaching and simply assume that it is the medical school's job. Many hospitals, not just teaching hospitals, receive money from a mechanism known as SIFT (Service Increment for Teaching) which is destined to meet the extra NHS costs associated with teaching medical and dental undergraduates. This currently runs at about £400 million a year and will be added in most cases to budgets which medical managers may feel are clinical budgets. In the past it was simply an item in the allocation, but as from 1999 allocation of this money will depend on a bottom up assessment of true costs of providing extra resources for undergraduate teaching.

In doing that unpicking the medical manager will need to cost items such as clinicians' undergraduate teaching sessions, the reduced number of patients seen in a teaching outpatients clinic, the provision of facilities for students to be taught in, the extra days of stay sometimes required so that patients can be taught on, etc. This is another one of the unhelpful time-consuming exercises in unpicking costs, a process which everyone resents as they see no likely benefit in it.

6.7 AUDIT, EVIDENCE-BASED MEDICINE AND MANAGED CARE

Thou wilt also learn one piece of Humility, viz. not to trust too much on thy own judgement.

(RICHARD WISEMAN, *Severall Chirurgicall Treatises 1676*)

A doctor's freedom to choose what he believes to be appropriate management for his patient is increasingly being modified. There are several drivers to change in this area; they have evolved over the last 10 years to the point where no clinician can claim ignorance and no one is uninvolved. They are sometimes represented as a progressive erosion of the clinician's priest-like individual power and may thus be a source of conflict between doctors and managers. It is important for the medical manager to understand the possible benefits and disbenefits of what is being done, as he is often the fulcrum about which the anxieties of clinicians and the aspirations of non-clinical managers rotate.

One might simplify this rolling revolution as follows; firstly there is a point of departure which is the historical *omnipotence of the clinician*. Even though as early as the time of Hippocrates the variability of practice between clinicians was understood as was the inappropriateness of some of what they did, and even though the development of the scientific method allowed some analysis of this, the principle of "the doctor knows best" generally held sway until this century. Only in the second half of this century has the notion of the individual doctor as the prime mover in a patient's care been seriously challenged. The challenge comes from two directions: firstly an appreciation that poor clinical outcomes might reflect faulty investigation, diagnosis or treatment and, secondly, that some investigations and treatments are more expensive than others and are often used inappropriately, i.e. there are both quality and cost aspects.

230

In the UK the response to this was the development of clinical audit as a peer review activity; either as a regular in-house exercise for the clinical team or nationally as in the Confidential Enquiry into Perioperative Deaths (CEPOD). In America overutilisation was the predominant theme and indeed was the predominant problem. The trend there was towards professional review with mandatory second opinion or professional reviewers to check that the investigations, treatment and lengths of stay remained within predefined limits. This was, and is, essentially a cost-containment exercise which merely substitutes the views of one doctor or group of doctors for that of another. The second opinion was presumed to be more educated or biddable about the cost–benefit ratio than the first opinion. What has gradually emerged, curiously late in history, is that doctors as a group may know better than others how to treat disease, but the individual doctor often does not know or apply the best management of disease—not through laziness or incompetence but simply through an inability to store, process and use the huge amounts of information that relate to disease and its management. Lawrence Weed has written about this,[28] and explicitly identifies the problem as "a misplaced faith in the unaided human mind," and that "until now we have believed that the best way to transmit knowledge from its source to its use in patient care is to first load the knowledge into human minds (the long and expensive education of professionals) and then expect those minds at great expense to apply the knowledge to those who need it. However there are enormous "voltage drops" along this transmission line for medical knowledge" and that therefore "good medical practice requires tools to extend the human mind's limited capacity to recall and process large numbers of relevant variables" and that "these tools should be kept up to date and used routinely—not in heads which are expensive to load and faulty in the attention and processing of knowledge". This would seem to be self evident, yet we continue to rely heavily on a high-quality, up-front education and accreditation processes. Even with continuing postgraduate medical education the level of knowledge of most individuals is probably inadequate for all but the highest level of hyperspeciality. Doctors in general are also handicapped by their difficulty in convincing themselves that they would accept external constraints on the untrammelled power of our own memories/ intuitions/skills to make crucial judgments about management. Hence the need for an audit process.

6.7.1 Audit

There is everything to be said in favour of the principles of clinical audit. All it asks is that clinicians critically review the results of their work on a regular basis, compare those results with those of others and if there are lessons to be drawn then change their practice. This describes the classic feedback loop of audit which turns into a repeating cycle or spiral to improve quality (Figure 6.7). These corrective feedback loops were thought to be the

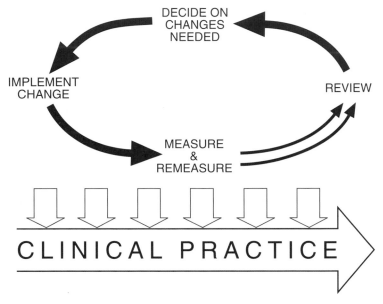

Figure 6.7   The audit cycle.

solution to the defects in our knowledge, but the audit process itself has proved to be a blunt and cumbersome tool. Audit, even aided by computers, clerks and audit officers, is only able to focus on a few problems at a time and experience shows that the feedback loop from measurement to changed practice to re-measurement is only rarely completed and, even when it is, it works very slowly. A National Audit Office report published in 1995[29] reviewed nearly 7000 audit projects and looked in detail at 1441 undertaken at eight trusts. They found lots of audit activity underway (as there should have been given the £61 million cost)—most had involved confirmation of the benefits of care, changes in the process of care or the production of guidelines. Evidence of specific benefit to patients was skimpy. Sadly only one in six projects had gone around the whole audit cycle and was being repeated.

It is customary to blame the failures of audit on the resistance of clinicians and their supposed unwillingness to have their shortcomings laid bare amongst their peers.[30] Years of attending "Deaths and Complications" meetings suggest that this is absolutely not the case. It seems more often that what has interfered with audit's ability to engage either our hearts or our minds is a frustration with the cumbersomeness of the audit process itself, the obviousness of the conclusions, and the powerlessness of the average clinician to change many of the causative defects in process. Audit has simply not made significantly more impact on day-to-day clinical practice than the normal evolution of professional knowledge would have made. So along came the armies of evidence-based medicine (EBM) whose cavalry have in most engagements quickly outflanked the dour and portly foot soldiers of the audit team.

The failures of audit

Audit as a core activity has been described as:

> a vicious circle, a noose to strangle any chance of it ever being a practical every-day tool ... a whole service industry has mushroomed around this fatal flower, and with every new blossom it becomes more and more remote from real practice and from the people who are actually doing the work.[31]

That is overstated; nevertheless a careful paper by Anthony Hopkins has analysed the reasons why audit has failed to win over the professionals.[32] He concluded that the problem is a conflict between clinical audit as a tool for education and professional development and its use for monitoring performance. He says in his summary:

> it is my belief that the simple methods sufficient to improve care in a local and low key way have been confused with the much more rigorous methods required to monitor contract performance and to begin to compare the performance of different hospital teams. A great deal of money has been spent on employing audit assistants with insufficient knowledge of the complexities of clinical measurement and yet who try to impose this insufficiency of knowledge on the informal methods of

233

directorate audit. No-one can criticise the NHS Executive for failing to provide financial resources to help first medical and then clinical audit, but this money was thrown at the problem without a sufficient research base in clinical audit, without sufficient attention to the social structures in hospitals and medical schools, and without sufficient recognition of the constructively critical faculties of health professionals.

i.e. good principle, shame about the practice!

One small consolation in this is that at least the NHS Executive appears to have realised that audit is not working and is supporting the Action on Clinical Audit project to explore the reasons for its failure.[33]

The ultimate irony for audit is that the benefits and cost effectiveness of audit have never themselves been properly audited; "we will never really know whether the national policy on clinical audit had a positive effect overall or whether the money could have been better spent. Audit will always be an act of faith".[34]

We should not leave audit on a negative note. Audit as an activity is growing up. The principle that guides it is sound, and slowly it is becoming better focused. One way of controlling it may be to commission specific audits from outside "suppliers" (this is called "outsourcing" if you want to use management speak). There are several purely commercial organisations who will now do this for a fee and even the Audit Department of the Royal College of Surgeons is now offering such a service. Of course the costs then immediately become explicit and in need of justifying; e.g. a Royal College of Surgeons audit of patient satisfaction costs between £3000 and £15 000. There are other ways. The British Association of Surgical Oncology for example with pharmaceutical company sponsorship, provides free software to breast units to enable them to collate their data in a format that allows anonymous comparisons with other units. The audit data is thus collected as part of the normal process of collecting clinical data with obvious cost benefits.

One thing that must be apparent even to those most irritated by the pedantic ways of audit is that much of the change that is occurring around us is indeed in need of audit. And not just management-driven change, even as radical and expensive a change in clinical practice as the widespread adoption of laparoscopic surgery has gone largely unaudited. Few of the predicted benefits of laparoscopic cholecystectomy seem to have accrued[35] and yet it

234

is a procedure which in prospect seemed very likely to have both health and economic benefits. Even so only 11 of 1500 publications on it in English since 1994 have been randomised trials.[36] As in so many areas there has been little evidence of the much needed clinical and managerial audit which should validate the implementation of new technology.

Confidentiality of audit records

A medical manager has not only a duty to ensure that audit is occurring effectively in her area but also must ensure that confidentiality is maintained for both patients or, "where appropriate", staff. Although it is claimed that clinical audit data is part of an educational process and its records not available to lawyers seeking to use them, this is, in fact, not so in reality. There is no specific protection for these records and there is no specific law relating to the disclosure of clinical audit information in the UK. A test case will be required to settle any legal issues which might arise.[37]

6.7.2 Evidence-based medicine

Nothing, of course, is new and for all that its acolytes claim that evidence-based medicine (EBM) is a unique event in medical history, it is not. There have been plenty of empiricist, epistemic and scientific doctors practising during the last thousand years who have managed to improve the quality of medical care through careful assessment of the available evidence. Anyone who feels that the current debate about EBM is new might usefully read Rangachari's paper "Evidence Based Medicine: Old French Wine with a New Canadian Label?",[38] in which he charts Pierre Louis' epistemic approach to the efficacy of blood letting in the management of disease and the positive and negative responses to his publications. All this was occurring in the first half of the nineteenth century. The clash then between the disciples of Louis' enthusiasm for the empirical approach versus the Gnostic clinicians' approach looking to the individual and human variability is exactly mirrored in papers of the 1990s. The philosophy underpinning EBM is simply the extension of a long historical thread that started when Newton and Descartes declared an overweening concern with observation, method, order and pattern to the exclusion of individuality.

The introduction and discussion sections of any clinical scientific publication have always aimed at educating the clinician to make "the conscientious, explicit and judicious use of current best evidence in making decisions about the care of individual patients", which in fact, is the definition of EBM given by Sackett.[39] The definition by Sackett is a clinician's definition, but much the same as Appleby's definition of EBM as "the rigorous evaluation of the effectiveness of health care interventions, common dissemination of the results of the evaluation and use of the findings to influence clinical practice".[40] Appleby's definition is subtly different and a manager's definition, but it is all good worthy stuff which arguably has been around for as long as there have been scientists and managers. What is, however, new, apart from a certain holier than thou gloss on the process, is that:

(1) The process of assessing the evidence has become more systematic and statistical and in the hands of statisticians rather than clinicians.

(2) The results of the analysis are deliberately refined into clinical guidelines.

(3) The process has been taken up (hijacked you might say) by public health doctors, managers, purchasers, and even the general public.

(4) Changes in information technology have allowed easier dissemination of the conclusions, e.g. the Cochrane database and the Internet.

(5) The process has also looked at structural issues, such as whether a higher flow of patients with a specific disease through a unit will produce better results.[41]

The central tenet of EBM is that a sophisticated analysis of the available data will yield a truth about the management of disease that can be the starting point for clinical guidelines which clinicians *ought* to use. The process even allows the guidelines to be annotated with an indication of the strength of the evidence that supports each recommendation. Levels of evidence quoted are:

Ia. A meta-analysis.
Ib. At least one controlled randomised trial.
II. At least one well-designed non-randomised trial.
III. Non-experimental descriptive studies such as comparative or case studies.

IV. "Respectable opinion".

It is a big leap from level I evidence, which is often scanty to a workable guideline, so the views of professional groups, of patients and of local users need to be integrated into any guidelines. This makes for a quasi-democratic product but not necessarily a clear one. Nevertheless, lots of guidelines are produced and in the process the scientific evidence on which we base our practice is sieved and graded and made available from sources such as the Cochrane database.

Crucially guidelines must include local input, as people are suspicious of guidelines defined and imposed by people they do not know. By analogy Dr Muir Gray likes to tell the story of Mary Baker who invented the first instant cake mix but found it did not sell until the powdered egg ingredient was omitted and the person making the cake contributed by breaking into the mix their own, real raw egg.[42]

Once guidelines are available they not only afford a core of reliable information to guide clinicians but they also help to improve communication with patients and other professionals who can all be working from the same data which is particularly important in the context of the discontinuous care now provided under the New Deal arrangements (Table 6.1). They improve risk management

Table 6.1 Checklist for desirable attributes when assessing guidelines

- Validity
- Cost effectiveness
- Reproducibility
- Reliability
- Patient and user involvement
- Clinical applicability
- Clinical flexibility
- Clarity
- Meticulous documentation
- Scheduled review date linked to audit

by identifying areas where training or supervision is needed. Guidelines in theory can improve the effective use of our resources. They can additionally identify research and audit needs. This all sounds optimistic but the guidelines have been shown genuinely to have these effects.[43]

The production of guidelines is, nevertheless, a laborious process and guidelines are not yet available for all eventualities, but we are getting there. A brave new era has dawned. The triumph of rationality and shared experience over ignorance and conservatism! Or is it? *Truth* as the French philosopher Michel Foucault observed is not something real and permanent but something "produced" by an elite as part of a "system of exclusion" of alternative options.

Problems with evidence-based medicine

There is much spoken and published criticism of EBM. Some just, some unjust based on a misunderstanding of what it's about. It is hardly surprising that there should be opposition; the term EBM itself implies that other medicine is not evidence based which is clearly not true, although EBM afficionados love to repeat the completely untested axiom that 90% of what doctors do has no scientific basis. What is primarily at stake is the legitimacy of the evidence advanced to support a decision about a patient's management. The quality of evidence which underpins EBM is on the surface exceptionally good, deliberately so, and thus its legitimacy would seem to be secure, but there is a danger in placing too much importance on the results of published clinical trials and then generalising them to the whole population. There is evidence to show that such published trials are biased in favour of interventional procedures and those with positive results. Multiple publications of the same data will also bias a result. Negative results tend not to be published,[44] as are studies looking at qualitative issues such as the attitudes and perceptions of patients, because these are not easy to grind in the statistical mill.[45] A population study must be clearly defined and tends to exclude the aged and those with comorbidity. The quest in EBM has been for "internally valid" evidence, i.e. scientifically pure, to the exclusion of "externally valid", i.e. generally applicable evidence.[46] More worrying, perhaps, are nagging anxieties about the crown jewel of EBM, the meta-analysis.[47] In the past we were warned about the dangers of combining disparate studies if we wished to have a believable result and combining disparate studies is what meta-analysis does. One study analysed meta-analyses for the sort of biases mentioned above and found bias in 38% of meta-analyses published in four leading journals.[48] Unfortunately there is no statistical way of resolving the problem of heterogeneity,[49] nevertheless a careful meta-analysis may indeed be the best means that we possess to assess the available data; its great danger is that its conclusions will be believed. The mechanics of the analysis are so opaque to the mere clinician or manager that what is concluded is likely to be taken as gospel even though it may quite simply be wrong. Le Lorier and his team in Montreal looked at instances where large randomised trials had addressed the same questions as previous meta-analyses. They found that in 35% of the instances studied the findings of the randomised study differed from those predicted by the meta-analysis![50] Hence a need not only for obsessional care about the processes of meta-analysis itself but also for great scepticism and even greater care when promulgating guidelines.[51,52]

Consensus and guidelines

The clinician unlike the basic scientist has to act even when knowledge is insufficient for a fuller informed decision. A "consensus" view under these circumstances can be achieved in only three ways: by compromise, by selection of an expert panel whose views conform, or by use of language that obscures differences.

When there are genuine differences of opinion in a review panel, compromise is the only way in which apparent unanimity can be obtained. The objection to describing the result as a consensus is that the term carries an authority that "compromise guidelines" would not. Bias in selection of a review panel is unlikely to be intentional, but nevertheless carries an important risk. Distinction in medical science reflects prevailing values and prejudices; the minority questioning voice may well not be selected, although it may belong to tomorrow's majority.

(EDITORIAL[51])

But we need guidelines

Whatever their shortcomings we need guidelines as one of the ways by which quality of care can be improved, if for no other reason than that doctors not only may not know what is current best treatment but may not know that they don't know![53] More importantly the use of publicised best practice is the surest way for the public to be assured that they are being properly treated. There are a large number of groups working to produce best practice guidelines, some national and some local. The NHS Executive attempts to keep a track of them and is a good source of current information through its "Guidelines Group", and in due

239

course through the activities of NICE the National Institute for Clinical Excellence. Central approval does not however remove the need for clinicians to assess guidelines themselves. The need for comprehensiveness and consensus leads to guidelines being sometimes vague ("might", "may", "could" featuring often) and the time taken for their completion and propagation can lead to them being out of date. For example, the Royal College of Surgeons of England's guidelines on hernia repair advocated the Shouldice technique, but was almost instantly rendered meaningless by the publication of the first large series showing the excellence of the Lichenstein mesh repair; information available to readers of the surgical journals but not available to those reading only the guidelines! But the most cogent criticism is that guidelines do not sit comfortably with the hurly-burly of daily clinical practice where doctors have to address not diagnoses but clinical problems, e.g. not angina but chest pain, and the guidelines are written for angina. Additionally, the guidelines are global and not specific and may not be appropriate for the old patient with concurrent problems or the GP as distinct from the hospital doctor. Lastly, they can subvert the cultural importance of the *art* of medicine, which involves understanding the whole patient from a physical, psychological and social perspective; treatment being based as much on experience and intuition as on a purely scientific approach. Twenty-five years ago Lord Platt wrote: "I am therefore somewhat concerned lest the extreme believer in the creed of scientific medicine should be bringing up a generation of doctors who can no longer trust their own observations or their judgement".[54] Many of us still share that anxiety:

> . . . the presence of reliable evidence does not ensure that better decisions will be made. Claims that evidence based medicine offers an improved method of decision making are difficult to evaluate because current practice is so poorly defined. Medical decision making draws upon a broad spectrum of knowledge—including scientific evidence, personal experience, personal biases and values, economic and political considerations, and philosophical principles (such as concern for justice), it is not always clear how practitioners integrate these factors into a final decision, but it seems unlikely that medicine will ever be entirely free of value judgements.
>
> (KERRIDGE *et al.*[55])

Does this matter? Well yes it can. If EBM were simply an exercise by doctors and academics for winnowing the mass of information that has accumulated then it would probably be safe. But the use of EBM has gone far beyond that. We may argue the scientific rights and wrongs of EBM but it is the inappropriate use of EBM for managerial purposes that is worrying, and it is here that the medical manager will need to ensure that sense prevails. Someone must not only judge the protocol itself, but also decide when a departure from protocol was not simply ignorance, and someone must have the wit to see when protocols are strangling innovation or humanity.

Rules are for the obedience of fools and the guidance of the wise.

(ANON)

Evidence-based medicine and the medical manager

In December 1993 an NHS Executive Letter (93/115) was issued covering "a developing initiative to integrate professional guidelines more effectively into the delivery of health care" and "to develop guidelines which will be useful in framing discussions between purchasers and providers on the development of service specifications and contract negotiations". EBM had moved from a clinical tool to a managerial one. That is not necessarily a bad thing, but the clinician in management now has a crucial role to ensure that non-clinicians wishing to use EBM guidelines understand their inadequacies and the potential dangers of a too rigid use of them. Dangers encapsulated, for example, in the notion that "clinical *effectiveness*" requires unstinting adherence to the guidelines, and that departure from them implies clinical *ineffectiveness*. EBM guidelines are, of course, valuable for suggesting an expected form of treatment with which to bring clinicians and units using out of date or less effective therapies up to date, but their unvarying use for every patient in a single unit carries hazards. The medical manager needs to ensure that clinical practice does not become "tyrannized by evidence"[56] such that everything is judged only against the guidelines and not seen in context.

On 23 September 1996 *The Times* reported that Chelsea and Westminster Health Authority had said "it would not pay for patients treated by any surgeon who failed to follow the protocols set out in its contract . . ." Their director of commissioning said,

241

"we have said we would not wish our patient to be treated by anyone who is not prepared to work to the best cancer protocols. My job is to ensure the contracts reinforce good practice." You can be certain that the medical manager had to sort out the clinicians' reactions to that and perhaps persuade the commissioner that no protocol exists which covers the needs of all patients.

I am not suggesting that the medical manager becomes Horatio On The Bridge holding back the barbarian hoards of EBM-crazed managers, simply that he be clear in his own mind of the benefits and dangers of EBM. He may also need to police the production of guidelines locally and to this end the NHS Good Practice Booklet *Clinical Guidelines* is helpful.[57] This publication also addresses the difficult issue of the legal position of guidelines and the anxiety that doctors have that departures from guidelines might weaken their position in any complaint or legal action against them. It is a complex area but the document concedes that the "Bolam test" will still apply and that the doctor's actions in any specific context are thus likely to be judged by whether a responsible body of peers would have acted in a similar way. The existence of professionally agreed guidelines will, however, certainly make it more difficult to justify departures from them, and it is expected that they will in time erode the Bolam principle which has guided medicolegal decisions for so many years. The Bolitho case may be the first step down that road. The Law Lords in deciding this appeal opined that the court has to be satisfied that "the exponents of a body of opinion relied on could demonstrate that such opinion had a logical basis".[58]

The clinical manager will also need to remember that too close a public adherence to guidelines can for many patients smack of medical authoritarianism and force them into the hands of alternative practitioners.

Lastly the medical manager needs to consider how guidelines can be moved from paper to practice. The implementation of guidelines is the implementation of change and the obstructions to change are usually people and their attitudes, sometimes also resources. Attitudes to change are more often conditioned by beliefs than by evidence and changing peoples' beliefs is difficult.[59]

Wary of the lack of audit the Department of Health has commissioned an "independent and rigorous appraisal service for clinical guidelines" from the Health Care Evaluation Unit at St George's Hospital Medical School and the King's Fund is assisting in some carefully monitored initiatives such as PACE (Promoting Action on Clinical Effectiveness).[60]

In summary
I have dwelt at length on EBM and managed care because I believe it is the single topic which will most tax the clinician in management over the next decade and thus all its ramifications should be thought through clearly. I would suggest that the medical manager needs to fix on the following ten points in relation to EBM:

Internally
(1) Be proactive: work towards the humane and rational application of EBM.
(2) Ensure guidelines are appropriate for local use.
(3) Ensure that the status of the guidelines is clear.
(4) If the organisation is officially to adopt them ensure that all concerned know this, agree it and have copies.
(5) In some instances you may need to ensure that the audit mechanism is engaged to assess the guidelines when they are in use.

Externally
(6) Ensure that purchasers understand the general and local limitations on the use of guidelines.
(7) Accept guidelines as part of a service specification only if the team involved agree and "let out" clauses are written into the service specification.
(8) Ensure that purchasers use EBM equitably adopting not only those guidelines that lead to cheaper care, but also those guidelines that lead to better but more expensive care.
(9) With centrally produced guidelines channel responses back to the place from whence they originated (professional group, royal college, etc.) to assist the process of continual modification and updating.
(10) Avoid the use of the word EBM as a mantra.

The words "EBM" and "audit" have become mantras for managers in hospitals just as "holistic medicine" and "shared care" have for GPs. There is danger that the simple repetition of the word in debate and documents will somehow confirm the worthiness of intent and that writing it in a contract will ensure purity and cheapness. Beware the word! Beware the fashion!

If the medical manager believes that the mechanical exercise of EBM is a valuable adjunct to defining best care and improving quality, then she may have to sell that to sceptical clinicians. Having accepted EBM as a constructive fact of life, she then runs the risk of turning to find the prospect of managed care advancing towards her as a darkening line on the horizon. It is currently abroad in the USA and is due to cross to the UK as surely as did Coca Cola and bubble gum.

6.7.3 Managed care

We have already seen how the doctor has willingly or otherwise given up his role of sole determiner of medical care, and we know that his relationship to the patient may subsequently have been damaged by what we might call resource-led care, in which the available resource is quantified and the care which he is allowed to offer is tailored to that quantity. With the help of EBM and his personal experience and commitment, the clinician can still define what he *believes* to be best for his patient, but may have to accept that circumstances prevent him from *delivering* it. The next stage is potentially more sinister for the clinician and his patient. In managed care the individual clinician's role in defining "best" treatment is usurped by the managed care process. Best treatment is then defined by an external group and protocols based on it are modulated by considerations of cost and resource availability. At its crudest this requires the doctor simply to make the diagnosis (and he may even be constrained in how he does this); thereafter the protocol takes over. That is managed care. The historic arrangement whereby the decision about how best to manage a patient's illness is decided between the clinician and the patient has been invaded by a process defined and managed by others who may or may not themselves be clinicians but who, nevertheless, do not have that primary relationship that the doctor has established between himself and the patient and which has always been judged to be the patient's safeguard. This is an environment where the stakes for doctors, patients and managers are high in human, professional and financial terms. In the USA where about 140 million people are covered by some sort of managed care arrangement the organisers of managed care are personally and corporately making enormous amounts of money and doctors are having their judgments and their incomes challenged as never

244

before. One might think that that side of it is not necessarily a risk in the UK, but the doctors' abilities to provide what they think are best for a particular patient will be eroded and we will need to come to terms with that. There will also be great temptations for future governments to abrogate responsibility for controlling an unmanageable and expensive health service to commercial organisations who will promise to control costs for a fee. The commercial sector in the UK is already sniffing around that particularly succulent prize.

There are a few experiments with managed care in Europe, most emphasising quality and efficiency from a patient's perspective. The French have introduced mandatory practice guidelines for a range of 147 common conditions. The guidelines, agreed professionally, were implemented from 1994 to 1995 and a system is in place to fine those who stray too far from them. The French are not notably acquiescent to bureaucracy, yet a review of the practice of 13 000 doctors led to only 75 of them being fined.[61] One hopes this reflects a close approximation of the guidelines to best clinical practice. Ensuring that the guidelines were written by professional groups uninfluenced by financial considerations may have been relevant. During this time the rate of increase of healthcare costs slowed but it is uncertain whether this was related; nevertheless in February 1998 the French government announced that as GP budgets had stayed within budget they would each receive a bonus of Fr9300 (£930). Many doctors and professional organisations objected that this was an unethical bribe for acquiescing to managed care and corrupted their professional independence. Many refused the bonus or donated it to charity (but were still taxed as if they had received it!). Although the French have been notably prescriptive and interventional in this area, it is predicted that managed care will generally be applied more subtly in Europe than it has been in America and that states will not for example have to enact laws making "drive-by mastectomies" (day-case mastectomy) illegal as the state of New York has had to. But before managed care arrives you would do well to read a series of three papers by Fairfield *et al.* in the BMJ.[62-64] To warn yourself of the dangers of managed care insofar as it represents a profit/savings led approach to healthcare you could also read "The two cultures and the health care revolution" by McArthur and Moore.[65] These very senior US authors identify 12 potential hazards from the shift to commercial managed care.

Some of these are currently only applicable in the USA but others are already apparent in the UK including downgrading of personnel, gagging clauses, neglect of research, and loss of choice.

The future of managed care

If purely professional considerations about the optimal care of patients are allowed predominance over financial and bureaucratic ones, managed care may merely be the careful application and facilitation of EBM and the smoothing of the process of delivering that care. Not all clinical care will be affected. The role of the medical manager will be central to the humanisation of managed care and to ensure that the hearts and minds of the clinical team are engaged. The clinical manager may need to expend a lot of negotiating effort explaining to purchasers that managed care is a professional exercise undertaken by professionals and not simply a further vehicle for bureaucratisation of the service. This is not a fanciful anxiety. One of the first sets of guidelines which have slipped into managed care (though it is not called that) has been the British Association of Surgical Oncologists' guidelines for the management of breast cancer. Purchasers have now turned this into a blueprint for managed care and are already expending large amounts of their own and others' time and energy in requiring documentation of each tiniest step in the protocol to ensure "compliance".

Found on the internet, quoted by Fairfield.[66]

> I used to be a doctor
> > Now I am a Health Care Provider
> I used to practice medicine
> > Now I function under a managed care system
> I used to have patients
> > Now I have a consumer list
> I used to diagnose
> > Now I am approved for one consultation
> I used to treat
> > Now I wait for authorization to provide care
> I used to have a successful people practice
> > Now I have a paper failure
> I used to spend time listening to my patients
> > Now I spend time justifying myself to the authorities

I used to have feelings
  Now I have an attitude
Now I don't know what I am.

6.8 MANAGING RESEARCH IN THE NHS
(by Nicol Thin, Director of Research, Guy's and
St Thomas' Hospital Trust)

The large range of operations which consist of amputating limbs
and extirpating organs admits of no direct verification of their
necessity. There is a fashion in operations as there is in sleeves
and shirts ... As a matter of fact, the rank and file of doctors
are no more scientific than their tailors.

(BERNARD SHAW: Preface to *A doctor's dilemma*)

6.8.1 Introduction

For many years the NHS supported research by a wide variety of
funding schemes which developed in a piecemeal fashion. It became
unclear whether the needs of the NHS were being met or even
addressed, and if resources were being targeted where they were
needed. An example was the research element of the Service
Increment for Teaching and Research. In 1990, in response to a
recommendation by a House of Lords select committee,[67] the
Government appointed a Director for Research and Development
(R&D) for the NHS, to place much more emphasis on research, to
give it more direction and to ensure better value for the considerable
amount of money being expended. At the same time there was a
desire to make the funding of research more explicit.

6.8.2 The NHS research and development strategy

NHS research and development (R&D) faces a challenge: to
maximise health gain from scientific developments while applying
research rigour to the problems confronting the NHS, the public
health and the social services. The director of R&D formulated an
NHS R&D strategy published in 1991.[68] The aim is to improve
the health of the nation by promoting a knowledge-based Health
Service in which clinical, managerial and policy decisions are
based on sound information from R&D findings and scientific
developments. The strategy is concerned with the development of

247

new practice, and rigorous evaluation and understanding of existing practice. It recognises that the health of the nation will gain from R&D and that the NHS should invest accordingly.

For NHS purposes, R&D is used to mean work which is designed to provide new knowledge:

- Potentially of value to those facing similar problems elsewhere (namely it is generalisable).
- Open to critical examination and accessible to all who could benefit from it (public dissemination).
- Relevant to the NHS.
- With a written protocol.
- Peer reviewed.
- Monitored.
- Approved by a research ethics committee where human subjects are involved.[69]

The NHS is concerned with clinical and health services research (formerly called operational research), namely work leading to new knowledge to benefit patients and other users of the service. The term research and development is used rather than research, to emphasise the importance of the Health Services research element. Health Services research brings together epidemiological, sociological, economic, and other analytical sciences in the study of health services and is usually concerned with relationships between need, demand, supply, use and outcome of health services. The aim is *evaluation*, particularly of structure, process, output and outcome, and includes users' views (adapted from Last[70]). An example might be a clinical drug trial where, in addition to clinical outcome (hitherto often the only outcome measure), the cost, cost–benefit and patient acceptability of different follow-up systems are evaluated. Users should have a say at all key stages of the R&D process. The NHS sees Health Services research as distinct from audit which is concerned with assessing practice against standards, correcting flaws and re-assessing to ensure improvement (closing the loop).

On the whole researchers like to undertake research which interests them and fits into their own programmes; the interests and aims of the sources of their funds may be forgotten once funding is obtained. Such activity may be of little general relevance. The new R&D agenda centres on the real knowledge required by the NHS as a managed service rather than a setting in which doctors practise medicine.

R&D funded by the NHS must conform to ten principles also referred to as the ten dimensions of assessment[3]:

(1) *Quality*—All work must be of high quality as judged by the prevailing professional standards.

(2) *Ethics*—All work must be ethical and approved by a research ethics committee when human subjects are involved.

(3) *Relevance, impact and importance*—R&D must be relevant to health gain in the short, medium or long term and contribute to the development of evidence-based policy and practice.

(4) *Primary care*—The NHS is keen to develop R&D in primary care. Wherever possible, there should be close collaboration in R&D between primary and secondary care in accordance with the NHS priority of achieving a primary care led service.

(5) *Partnership*—The greatest overall gain will flow from cooperation between NHS purchasers and providers, universities, other R&D funders including industry and local authorities.

(6) *Strategy*—R&D and its funding must have a strategy which integrates with an overall strategy. Those bidding for NHS R&D funds are expected to demonstrate an R&D strategy or the ability to develop one.

(7) *Appropriate disciplinary mix*—R&D should involve and promote the most appropriate mix of skills and expertise. The NHS emphasises the value of all healthcare professionals in R&D.

(8) *Integration with other NHS activities*—R&D and its funding should always integrate with the many other activities within the NHS.

(9) *Cost*—Funds must be used as efficiently as possible.

(10) *Management*—Robust, transparent, effective management of R&D funds must be in place.

Although this is a list of worthy criteria, it is perhaps somewhat idealistic. For better or worse it runs the risk of inhibiting just the kind of spontaneous, low-technology "ruler and string" research which traditionally was a strength of British research sometimes leading to important achievements. The discovery of penicillin might be regarded as an example. Arguably, the day for that sort of activity has passed and the commissioning and practice of R&D now needs to be more formal and transparent.

6.8.3 NHS R&D structures and funding streams

NHS funding for R&D comes in a variety of streams. The following description applies to England, but Scotland, Wales and Northern Ireland have similar arrangements. Most funds come from the NHS Levy on health authorities which the NHS Executive retains and subsequently redistributes for R&D. In total this is slightly less than 1.5% of the total spending on the NHS. This funding is sometimes referred to as Culyer Funding after Professor Anthony Culyer, whose name was attached to the report recommending this new structure for NHS R&D funding.[71] The Levy is divided into two budgets.[72]

Budget 1 of the NHS Levy—R&D support funding for NHS providers

This funding comprises approximately 82% of the Levy. It is designed to meet the additional *clinical* costs of undertaking clinical research funded by the major non-commercial research funders, namely, the MRC and other research councils, the Wellcome Trust and other members of the Association of Medical Research Charities, the NHS, the Department of Health and other government departments, and the European Union. In addition this funding meets the infrastructure costs of undertaking clinical and health services research not covered from other sources, namely pre-protocol and own account research. The funding is disbursed in two forms.

Portfolio Funding is intended for providers with a reasonably predictable flow of external funding and large enough to take a strategic approach to managing their R&D. It is a block grant to meet all providers' relevant R&D support costs and providers have some flexibility in switching funds from one activity to another within their organisation. This is the sort of block grant that teaching hospitals have traditionally enjoyed.

Task Linked Funding is directly linked to tasks or areas of activity and is usually granted to smaller providers of primary or secondary care. Grants are made for 3 or 4 years.

This Support Funding does *not* support commercially funded projects. It is important for providers to obtain grants from the non-commercial sources if they wish to maintain their Support Funding. It is providers who bid for Support Funding, not individuals.

Budget 2 of the NHS Levy—the NHS R&D programme

This takes approximately 18% of the Levy and allows the NHS to commission and fund programmes and projects perceived to be priorities for the organisation itself. Central and regional programmes are funded.

Central programmes include the UK Cochrane Centre, the NHS Centre for Reviews and Dissemination, and the Health Technology Assessment Programme. In the budget allocation process, both the individual programme organisers and the NHS Executive call for bids; those interested must remain aware of the current and probable future priorities within the service so they can respond in a timely fashion to calls for submissions. These calls to bid are advertised in the medical press and by the NHS Executive regional offices directly to providers. The bids may be for original work, often called "primary research", or reviews, also called "secondary research".

Regional programmes fund priorities identified by NHS Executive regional offices. Currently various forms of funding are available, including project grants for sums up to £80 000 over 1 or 2 years. Fellowships and bursaries provide research opportunities and formal training for NHS staff who have a potential to develop themselves as researchers. Fellowships are normally for 2 years and cover a salary up to £30 000 per year, project expenses up to £5000, the registration fee for a higher degree and the cost of up to three training courses at a maximum £1500 each. Bursaries with a current maximum of £6000 support NHS staff and primary care contractors for 1 or 2 years to develop skills which will enable them to undertake research of direct importance to their work.

It is important that requests for bids accurately and clearly describe what is wanted; for success bidders must meticulously follow the requirements stated in the bid announcement. Before submitting a bid, it is wise to have a preliminary discussion with the central or regional office and their statistics unit. Grant holders are closely monitored.

6.8.4 Non-commercial research funds

Sources of these funds include the MRC and other research councils, the Wellcome Trust and other members of the Association of Medical Research Charities, the NHS, the Department of Health and other government departments, and the European Union.

These advertise their grants in the medical press. Most large providers will also have a system to circulate details to interested researchers within their organisation. It is important to follow the directions for bidding with care. Inexperienced researchers should obtain advice in preparing their bid from experienced and successful colleagues. Many funding organisations concentrate their grants within specific areas, so researchers should discover the interests of each organisation and submit bids accordingly. It is wise, especially when applying for large grants, to have informal discussions with funders before bidding.

6.8.5 Commercial research funds

This is the funding provided by industry to support clinical trials of new drugs, devices, and instruments. This funding must support *all* the costs of the work involved. Increasingly clinical trials organisations are working with manufacturers and providers to encourage and promote clinical trial work. Individuals within trusts do not bid competitively to undertake trials in the same manner that is required by the NHS, research trusts, and charities. Collaborations develop through personal contacts made with representatives of firms when they visit providers, or at medical meetings and conferences. Most drug trials are multicentre and many are multinational; this means a loss of ownership for individual departments and researchers, but this work is often an important source of income for departments which most are eager to maximise.

6.8.6 Provider R&D strategies

Just as the NHS has an R&D strategy, it is important for providers who are to be successful in obtaining funds from the NHS and other major research funders to have an R&D strategy. This involves assessing the organisation's strengths, interests and potentials, and those of its partners such as collaborating universities, purchasers and other providers including primary care. It may be wise for providers to bring together some of their R&D strengths in themes or groups which may be virtual or real. At the same time to maintain vibrant, progressive and innovative R&D, new researchers and topics must be encouraged. In developing a strategy all researchers should have an opportunity to contribute to a

252

transparent process within their own organisations so they can all have a sense of ownership. The strategy should be forward looking and revised at least once a year.

6.8.7 The role of medical managers in R&D

R&D is no longer an option in the NHS; it is a core function. Although some of the above may seem a little daunting, everyone working in the service should feel encouraged and excited to be part of an organisation that is so progressive and eager to improve services through R&D. Medical managers have considerable responsibilities relating to R&D although some of the work may be delegated.

Manager's role in creating the infrastructure for R&D
Whether in small or large providers, medical managers should encourage R&D and create an environment and ethos for R&D to flourish. They must understand that it is part of their organisation's function to ensure that an adequate infrastructure is in place, including access to libraries, information technology and study leave. In smaller organisations there may be only a few small projects; here the medical manager's major role may be to ensure that practice is evidence based and that all healthcare professionals keep up to date with R&D findings from elsewhere in the service.

Despite all the pressures throughout the organisation, time must be made available for R&D. Providers must ensure the involvement of nurses, midwives and all professionals allied to medicine as well as doctors and dentists, and make R&D training available to all staff. Everyone should understand the importance of clinical and Health Services research; the latter should be included in all projects wherever possible. Furthermore, R&D findings must be translated into practice, a previously neglected and difficult area, and practice evaluated. Managers have a special role in this area which overlaps with audit and evidence-based medicine as discussed earlier (section 6.7.2). Clinicians are usually well informed, enthusiastic and pragmatic but wary when it comes to change.

Managers should ensure that university and other purchaser and provider collaborations are in place where appropriate, and that R&D is multidisciplinary involving other professionals as well as doctors and dentists. For those in secondary care, R&D should

253

link with primary and community care wherever relevant. For those in the community, collaborations with other community purchasers and providers as well as secondary care providers, and academic bodies should be considered.

Medical managers should be aware of the R&D projects already underway in their area of responsibility, to ensure, for example, that the activity is fully funded. Clinical managers should collaborate with financial and administrative managers to ensure that robust transparent accounting systems are in place.

Managerial involvement in the R&D process

Medical managers should be involved at all stages of R&D, from preliminary discussion, pre-protocol work, protocol development, research ethics committee approval, bidding for funds, encouraging the actual work at all stages, and ensuring findings are reported, whether by writing a report for the regional office, placing a summary on the NHS internet, publishing in a peer-reviewed journal or giving presentations at local, regional or international meetings. The managerial involvement of doctors in this may be intense if, for instance, a clinician has been appointed specifically to manage research. But even when R&D is occurring as a minor part of a clinical directorate's overall work, the clinical director must understand and be associated with research activity so it does not become an unregarded add-on activity at the margin.

Clinical managers have another major role in the R&D process. There is a lack of basic knowledge required to inform management decisions in the NHS. Managers need to identify gaps in this knowledge base and initiate projects to provide information to fill these gaps.

Lines of responsibility

There must be a line of responsibility for R&D from clinical departments up through directorates to the medical director. The NHS Executive expect a board member to have a responsibility for R&D, at least in the larger providers. Many larger providers have appointed staff to coordinate R&D and respond to the demands made by the NHS. This will include collaborating with the National Research Register which in due course it is hoped will hold details of all projects and be available for consultation by all researchers to complement library searches and the Cochrane and other databases. In the future there may be a need to collaborate with other central bodies in the NHS such as the proposed National Institute for Clinical Excellence.[73]

6.8.8 Conclusion

Medical managers must foster R&D by providing the infrastructure and encouraging individuals. Although the culture of R&D adds to already heavy workloads at a time of rapid change throughout the NHS, there are exciting opportunities to grasp especially for NHS Executive funding for Health Services research across the primary secondary care interface to smooth it into a continuum, and within the community. With the culture of user-orientated R&D improving the evidence base for practice in all its facets, the NHS can look forward to a stimulating future in the new millennium. As has been noted elsewhere in this book, it is vital that doctors engage in the process of managing and do not simply dismiss it as a bureaucratic sideline.

6.9 COMPLAINTS

Although we are healthier than we have ever been we are more anxious about our health than any past generation, in addition our old notions of misadventure, Acts of God and sheer bad luck have been cast aside and replaced by an unmodulated culture of blame. Health is to be perceived as a right, a natural state even, and if "Medicine" and "The World Around Us" does not keep us healthy then someone must be to blame.[74] It is hardly surprising therefore that some patients complain. In fact, the number who do so formally is very, very few even in the current epidemic of complaint. In 1996–97 the hospital and community health services received 93 000 written complaints which represents a tiny fraction of the millions of contacts during the year. A Gallup survey commissioned by *The Daily Telegraph* in 1998 showed that 46% of respondents had used the NHS in the previous 3 months and 91% were satisfied with their treatment.[75] The small number of complainants, the fact that some of them are readily seen to be merely vexatious, plus the hurt felt by staff when a complaint is received, can lead to a culture of ignoring complaints or at least of not taking them seriously. That is wrong; all the pundits say it is wrong and detailed recommendations and protocols exist for dealing with complaints. More of that later. But first for the sceptic just a moment's reflection

255

on why most of us hate complaints; maybe the better to understand the pattern of our response.

I suspect the great majority of doctors, nurses and others in the Health Service feel that they are doing the best that they can with inadequate resources in difficult circumstances. The patients traditionally shared this ethic as if we were all still in the Blitz together; we did not like it but we would do our best together. The patient who complains that her bed in the air-raid shelter is too lumpy or there is plaster dust in her tea clearly does not share the ethic and when there is personal spite as well, "*you* allowed my bed to get lumpy", "*you* did nothing to stop plaster dust getting in my tea", then staff feel doubly aggrieved. I have trivialised the example to make a point. Complainants feel their complaints passionately but the personal consequences for staff involved in a complaint can be very significant. Doctors have killed themselves because of the stress of a long-running complaints process, many others say it is a factor in seeking early retirement. Nurses, clerks and others simply leave the service. I would say there is one important—very important—message from this. It is this. Every complaint has the capacity not only to inform staff for the purposes of improving the service (the Official view) but also has the capacity to harm, demoralise and discourage them. The harm is sometimes proportionally many times greater than the complaint would seem to merit. Protocols for handling complaints must reflect this. The current practice of assuming the patient/customer is always right is erroneous in the context of a nationalised health service. Many complaints are ill founded or the errors they report unavoidable. I believe that where the staff involved are not at fault they must be supported and defended. This may even involve defending a case legally at greater cost than simply pretending to be wrong and making a quicker and cheaper settlement. If we cherish our staff as much as our patients we owe them this.

Now that we have got that off our chest, back to the handling of complaints.

6.9.1 The culture of complaint

People have always complained about poor service, we all do it, but the recent rise in the numbers of complaints about healthcare seems to have coincided with the arrival of "The Patient's Charter". You can, if you wish, view the Patient's Charter as the Great Leap

Forward—a cultural revolution—insofar as it tried to tighten up a perceived, lackadaisical attitude to quality in the public services. A cynic's retort might be that it was simply a way of trying to improve a few, high-profile, measurable items at no cost while shifting the blame for failure in the Health Service onto the front-line staff. Both interpretations can be true. What is also true is that Charter standards as well as distorting the way healthcare is delivered mandated patients to complain. The complaints are, interestingly, not just about failures to meet Charter standards, but a whole variety of other issues. The one-way nature of complaints reflects the untrammelled individualism, the *"liberalisme sauvage"* set in motion by Margaret Thatcher and her successors, but happily we are promised a new Patient's Charter which will stress the responsibilities of patients as well as their rights.

6.9.2 Facing up to complaints

In spite of everything I have said thus far most complaints are genuine and reflect a patient's real unhappiness with what has happened. That unhappiness needs treating and in the process much may be learnt about the defective processes and personalities within the organisation. What should we do? *Firstly* try to avoid situations where problems mature into complaints. This requires the people at the scene to render first aid. It needs honesty and forthrightness at the time of a problem and a preparedness to talk it through with the patient. You may feel that this is a natural response for staff, but it is not reliably so and in our trust we found it necessary to issue a card to all staff (Figure 6.8). This attracted some derision but appears to have had a beneficial effect. Where a complaint has actually been made in writing it should be documented, dealt with through a formal process whose principles were laid out in the Wilson report.

6.9.3 Principles of managing complaints

The Secretary of State has issued directions and regulations about the management of complaints which are based on the "Hospital Complaints Procedure Act 1985". Although it is an old act the tightening up of procedures is more recent. The new procedures came into effect on 1 April 1996 to obtain certain key objectives.

257

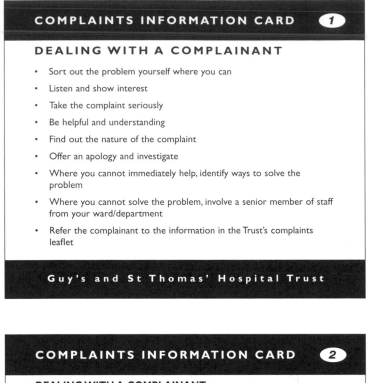

COMPLAINTS INFORMATION CARD ①

DEALING WITH A COMPLAINANT

- Sort out the problem yourself where you can
- Listen and show interest
- Take the complaint seriously
- Be helpful and understanding
- Find out the nature of the complaint
- Offer an apology and investigate
- Where you cannot immediately help, identify ways to solve the problem
- Where you cannot solve the problem, involve a senior member of staff from your ward/department
- Refer the complainant to the information in the Trust's complaints leaflet

Guy's and St Thomas' Hospital Trust

COMPLAINTS INFORMATION CARD ②

DEALING WITH A COMPLAINANT

Where you cannot solve the problem do involve a senior member of staff or the Quality Directorate but do not just shuttle the complaint around.

TIME SCALE FOR DEALING WITH COMPLAINTS

- Written complaints must be acknowledged within two days of receipt
- Complaints should be resolved and the complainant have received a full response within 28 days of receipt

CONFIDENTIALITY

- All patients are entitled to absolute confidentiality
- Staff should limit the discussions of complaints to those staff immediately concerned and treat all complaints as confidential

For help and advice in complaints handling contact:
The Directorate of Quality & Nursing
Guy's Tel 0171 955 4552   St Thomas' Tel 0171 922 8238

Guy's and St Thomas' Hospital Trust

Figure 6.8   Laminated card for staff, reminding them how to deal with complaints.

- Ease of access to the system for complaints.
- A simple, rapid, open process common to all parts of the NHS.
- Fairness for complainants and staff alike.
- Lessons from complaints to be used to improve patient services.
- Investigation of complaints to be entirely separate from any subsequent disciplinary proceedings.

Simple comments and complaints are sometimes resolved simply by there being an easy mechanism for making them. The act of complaining resolves the problem and informs the organisation of weak points and potential fracture lines which may need attention. A ready supply of forms on which complaints can be made eases this process though the dispenser boxes need to be kept topped up; an empty box exacerbates the problem!

Major complaints
If they are to be acted upon formal complaints must be made by patients over the age of 16 who have a normal mental capacity, though other people may complain on the patient's behalf with the patient's written authority. Complaints in general must be made within 6 months of the event complained about or from the moment at which the patient realised there had been a problem. These time limits can exceptionally be extended.

Essentially the process of dealing with complaints goes through three quite separate stages:

(A) Local resolution.
(B) Independent review.
(C) Appeal to the Health Service Ombudsman.

A. Local resolution
Every effort must be made to resolve complaints promptly and locally. Ideally this is in the form of an immediate informal response by the person who receives the complaint, and if that does not satisfy the complainant then there should be a speedy and open investigation; this is normally undertaken by specially appointed complaints staff skilled in not only laying their hands on the details and interpreting them, but also mediating. Experience shows that 75% of grievances can be resolved promptly in this way if the process is truly open and sympathetic. What must *not* happen is that the complainant is put down, ignored, side-lined or, at the

259

very worst, has it implied that a complaint will influence the quality of care that he receives in future. If the complaint is justified someone, ideally a person close to the event, should be prepared to make a proper apology for what has happened. Doctors are often worried about doing this for fear it will imply liability, but it does not. The important thing is that if an apology is due it should be given. It is the Department of Health's intention that most oral complaints should be resolved at the time or within two working days.

Written complaints must all culminate in a response in writing from the chief executive of the health authority or trust. Some written complaints are multifaceted and require quite careful investigation of the clinical circumstances, the obtaining of statements from clinicians and a direct approach to clinicians and other staff to ask their views on what happened. All those responses need to be put together and a reply constructed which the chief executive can then sign and send out to the patient. The Department of Health intends that this should always be completed within a month. That sounds a long time and it probably seems so for the complainant, but it is exceptionally difficult to get together the notes of a complicated case and the views of clinicians whom we have noted earlier will be disheartened and/ or irritated by the complaint. It is important to remember that the regulations require that any response that refers to matters of clinical judgment must be agreed by the practitioner before it is sent out.

If the complainant is dissatisfied with the outcome of "local resolution" to an oral or written complaint, then they may request an independent review.

B. Independent review

If a complainant asks for an independent review that does not invariably entitle them to have such a review. Reviews are difficult and time consuming and it is critical that requests for them are properly assessed. Regulations allow this insofar as such requests are first looked at by a "convenor". This will be a non-executive or lay director of the trust or health authority. It is a difficult task. The convenor, who by definition has no medical knowledge, has to try to obtain a comprehensive picture of what has happened, not only in relation to the events themselves, but also to find out whether the local resolution procedures were properly carried through. In doing this the convenor may need to take independent advice, usually clinical from outside or inside the trust or health authority. The convenor must discover whether legal proceedings are actually underway or threatened. The convenor at the end of this assessment can decide that:

- The local resolution process needs more time and effort put into it and is worth pursuing further.
- The local resolution adequately answered the complaint and that there are no grounds for proceeding to an independent review.
- A review should not proceed because legal proceedings are underway.
- An independent review should be undertaken.

For an independent review a "panel" is set up with a lay chairperson who is chosen from a regional list held by the Secretary of State. The panel consists of three people:

- The chairperson.
- The convenor.
- Another lay person.

The chairperson has the discretion about how the panel goes about its business but is required to arrange things within the following rules:

(1) The proceedings must be confidential.
(2) The panel must have access to all records about the handling of the complaint so far.
(3) If the complaint is clinically based the panel must have access to the relevant part of the clinical record.
(4) The panel must give the complainant and the practitioner complained against a reasonable opportunity to express their views in writing or verbally.
(5) The panel should not operate in a confrontational or legalistic way, as its intention is solely to establish the facts. No legal representation of any party is allowed.
(6) Complainants may be accompanied by an adviser, for example, from the Community Health Council. Similarly practitioners may be accompanied by a representative from their professional organisation or other "friends". Advisers and friends may only contribute to the proceedings with the approval of the chairperson.

Once the panel has accumulated the information about the case it must, if it relates to clinical matters, appoint at least two external

261

independent assessors. These assessors in turn will have access to all the records and may interview or even examine the patient. They do not then write a report, they merely submit their observations to the lay panel.

When all the facts and the clinical opinions have been gathered, the panel is required to produce a final report, a copy of which is sent to the complainant, the practitioners concerned and the chief executive. The chief executive will then decide whether any action needs to be taken and advise the complainant of his decision. He is additionally required to advise the complainant that if they are still dissatisfied they may take their grievance to the Health Service Ombudsman. All this should take no more than 3 months; a timescale which is often difficult to meet.

Once the panel has produced its report that stage of the process has been completed and cannot be repeated. The only avenue open to the continuing complainant is the Ombudsman or the law.

C. Appeal to the Health Service Ombudsman

If a complainant has exhausted the local resolution and independent review process and still feels unsatisfied, she can appeal to the Health Service Ombudsman. The Ombudsman will review all the paperwork which has been generated by the local resolution and independent review processes and may appoint his own independent advice. If the matter is related to clinical judgment, then he is required to have the assistance of two specialist assessors. If the Ombudsman decides to go ahead one of his staff will interview the party involved and, in due course, produce a final report which must be sent to the chief executive of the organisation involved for action, for comments or for recommendations. The Ombudsman may also make his own recommendations about disciplinary action in relation to clinicians and other practitioners or may suggest that a reference is made to the GMC or other regulatory body. The Ombudsman does not, himself, have any disciplinary powers.

It is important for clinicians to understand that they also have the right of appeal to the Ombudsman if they feel that the local resolution or, more likely, the independent review process has led to them "suffering hardship or injustice", and obviously in any such appeal they would want to seek the assistance of their medical defence organisation.

Problems with the new system

Although the new complaints system seems straightforward and equable to all parties, there has been much dissatisfaction particularly in relation to the independent review stage. Those who have experienced it have not infrequently reported that the panel has been unsympathetic, confrontational and sometimes straightforwardly aggressive, or that it has led to the initiation of disciplinary procedures against staff or their suspension without "due process". Even though these problems seem to arise from the overreliance on lay persons for coming to a judgment (and one would think it would make it more likely that claimants would be satisfied), evidence is that they are frequently not satisfied by the panel process if it does not go in their favour. The NHS Trust Federation has reviewed the workings of the new process and has not found evidence of difficulty in meeting the timescales. Anxieties have been expressed about the difficulty of recruiting non-executive directors to be assessors or to participate in panels. The whole business of the panel was found to be too time consuming, too bureaucratic and had no way of dealing with vexatious complainants. To the best of my knowledge there are no immediate plans to modify the process and in fairness it probably needs a longer trial.

Certainly it seems at present that the failure of the independent review process may partly explain the rise in complaints to the NHS Ombudsman, who received 2219 complaints in 1996/97, a rise of 24% over the previous year but nevertheless tiny in relation to the total volume of NHS business.

Complaints that turn into litigation

However carefully you deal with a complaint the outcome often seems to be unsatisfactory for the complainant who rarely falls on the complaints officer's neck thanking her for resolving the problem. The complainant who only wants to find out what happened may be content simply with the information, but the aggrieved complainant often wants more and the mollifying tone of the letter from the complaints officer or chief executive who acts as an intermediary between those involved and the complainant may be the very agent that further irritates the complainant who becomes more angry rather than less. Such a complainant may not even understand his own motives; for example, when the complainant is the relative of someone who has died the complaint may be an expression of the anger of grief inappropriately expressed. Not

263

infrequently the complainant wants not an explanation but somehow to punish the system for a real or imaginary hurt sustained. The sanitised apology does not suffice, she wants floggings, heads on poles, long periods of incarceration in dank dungeons with rats. But these are no longer open to her, so the embittered complainant passes from process to process, from complaints officer to panel to Ombudsman to their MP and then eventually to law using up inordinate amounts of staff time and emotional energy. This may be a happy reflection on the options of the population to pursue a just solution, but it is a very unwelcome process for most hospitals.

Some complainants will go straight to a solicitor without even stopping off to make a verbal complaint in the hospital. Whatever the route the end point of threatened or actual litigation is important for the institution. The costs both of defending or of losing a case will fall on the institution and such claims are rising and form a significant part of the budget. In 1998 the Medical Defence Union reported a 50% rise in the cost of claims for 1997 over 1995. Single claims can be enormous, and in the context of the NHS may be an inappropriate way to spend the nation's resources. A brain-damaged baby judged to be so because of defective hospital care can take a million pounds out of the hospital's budget and the hospital still needs to care for the child under the NHS. A child similarly brain damaged by some other misadventure is similarly cared for but gets nothing. Litigation lawyers remind us that claims are not about to reach a ceiling in terms of absolute numbers. It has been said that only 1 in 12 of those who have a good case for litigation actually proceed. This is obviously a source of distress to lawyers who see missed opportunities for enrichment, but it has helped to keep down the overall cost to the Health Service which is 0–4% of the total health expenditure, and currently about £200 million per year.

The reasons why most complaints do not go to law is probably nothing to do with the success of the internal complaints, but simply the difficulties of it. Going to law is almost solely the privilege of the legally aided. Access to legal aid appears to be quite easy for those whom a means test finds eligible. The decision as to whether to grant legal aid is based on the advice of the applicant's lawyers who have, of course, a direct financial interest in advancing the claim, and tend to take little expert medical advice before putting forward the case for legal aid. The numbers of

personal injury cases supported by legal aid have thus risen from
5000 to 16 000 over the last 10 years. A measure of the excessive
ease with which legal aid is obtained in medical negligence cases
is the low success rate of such actions. Only 17% of the 12 576
legally aided medical negligence cases closed in the year to 1 April
1996 were successful. The success rate in cases for other forms of
personal injury such as accidents at work is 85–90%. The whole
process is very protracted, the average time from the issue of
proceedings to conclusion is 6 years and 5 months.

The medical manager should be aware of three changes that will
affect this current practice over the next 10 years:

(A) Conditional/contingency fees ("no win, no fee").
(B) The recommendations of the Woolf Report.
(C) Changes in the regulations relating to the granting of legal
     aid.

A. No win, no fee
The legislation to allow lawyers and their clients to come to
conditional agreements about fees—the fee being conditional on
the outcome of the case—came into effect in July 1995. There
was alarm that this would allow the "ambulance chasing" and
speculative litigation common in the USA to appear in the UK.
Fortunately, there are other differences in the law between the UK
and the USA which make this unlikely. In the USA the plaintiff
and the defendant pay their own costs regardless of the outcome,
whereas in the UK the loser must pay the other party's costs. The
option, therefore, of not having to pay your lawyer if you lose does
not guarantee a risk fee exercise for the plaintiff, although in theory
it is possible to *insure* for the other party's costs if you lose, the
uncertain outcomes of medical litigation are expected to make this
prohibitively expensive. The no win, no fee arrangement also puts
greater pressure on the plaintiff's solicitor to check that the case
is worth pursuing, and that pressure is much greater than it is in
legally aided cases. Overall the system will probably reduce rather
than increase the number of vexatious and speculative claims.[76]
Doctors in the UK also retain the continuing privilege of the
application of the "Bolam Test". The Bolam Test is applied by a
judge to claims that a doctor was negligent and requires him to
accept a defence that a responsible body of practitioners trained
in the same specialty would have acted similarly.[77,78] Although the

265

Bolitho Case of 1997 if cited in future could require that medical experts' views as well as reflecting sound medical practice must demonstrate that they have considered the comparative risks and benefits of any action.[58]

B. The Woolf Report[79]

The Woolf Report reviewed the whole of the civil justice system in England and Wales and recommended radical change. Medical negligence litigation did not escape his attentions because he considered most cases currently to be unduly long, complex, and expensive. In a sample of medical negligence cases that his commission reviewed they found the average time from first contact with a lawyer to resolution was 65 months, and for claims worth less than £12 500 the legal costs of just one side averaged 137% of the claim's value! Lord Woolf also found that unmeritorious cases were pursued for too long and the degree of lack of cooperation and mutual suspicion was greater than in any other class of litigation.[80]

The recommendations of the report have been summarised as follows:

(1) Greater effort at prevention and early resolution of disputes. As steps towards this he recommended that medical record keeping should be better, the procedures for local resolution of problems should be clearer and that there should be more use of mediation with jointly instructed experts where possible and a greater use of experts' meetings. Overall though he recommended a more sparing use of experts.

(2) An improved summary disposal procedure to weed out weak claims and weak defences.

(3) The introduction of a system of plaintiff "offers to settle" with sanctions where a defendant unreasonably refused to cooperate.

(4) Claims of £10 000 or less to be handled by a slimmed-down procedure with a limited range of legal processes conforming to tightly controlled timetables and costs.

(5) Large and complex claims to be handled by a "multi-track" process where the management of each case legally is decided by the courts themselves rather than by lawyers.

Much of this was welcomed although there is considerable scepticism about the prospect of only a single medical expert being involved in some cases. The final outcome of the Woolf Report is yet to be determined but it would be prudent for medical managers to follow the arguments and the alternative proposals through as they evolve.[81] One early government response has been to propose limiting the choice of solicitors who are allowed to take on legally aided work in this area.

A number of pilot schemes are underway. In the meantime, in response to EL (96) 11 which outlines policy for handling clinical negligence and personal injury litigation, most Health Service organisations should have established a clear set of rules within their organisation.

C. Changes to legal aid legislation

The costs of legal aid are rising annually and are a headache for the government. Recent changes to the rules so as to reduce access to legal aid excluded medical negligence cases. Curiously instead of addressing the problems within the system the Secretary of Health and the Lord Chancellor merely put their efforts into "Naming and Shaming" those lawyers who are earning most from the system, which moved the debate forward not at all. The medical manager should therefore live in the continued expectation of protracted, frustrating and often futile combats with the legal advisers of the legally aided.

References

1 Barnes P. In: Simpson J, Smith R, eds. *Management for Doctors*. London: BMJ Publishing Group, 1995, pp. 45–54.
2 Webb AK, Hanley SP. The conflict in transferring a cystic fibrosis specialist service between two hospitals in Manchester. *Br Med J* 1997; **315**:1009–11.
3 Goddard M, Ferguson B. *Mergers in the NHS*. London: Nuffield Trust, 1997, p. 85.
4 Kennedy I *et al*. Dear Mr Dobson. *Br Med J* 1997;**315**:147.
5 Klein R. *Br Med J* 1996;**314**:508.
6 Thornton S. The case of Child B—reflections of a chief executive. *Br Med J* 1997;**314**:1838–9.
7 Maynard A. Rationing health care. *Br Med J* 1996;**313**:1499.
8 Klein R. Priorities and rationing. Pragmatism or principles? *Br Med J* 1995;**311**:761–2.
9 New B, ed. *Rationing; talk and action in health care*. London: BMJ Publishing Group, 1997.
10 Smith R. Rationing health care. Moving the debate forwards. *Br Med J* 1996;**312**:1553–4

11 Ham C, Honigsbaum F, Thompson D. Priority setting for health care. In: Oakley A, Williams AS, eds. *The Politics of the Welfare State*. London: UCL Press, 1994, pp. 98–126.

12 Smith R. Being creative about rationing. *Br Med J* 1996;**312**:391–2.

13 Weale. Rationing health care. *Br Med J* 1998;**316**:410.

14 Gillam S, Penceon D. Managing demand in general practice. *Br Med J* 1998;**316**:1895–8.

15 Wyatt JC. Hospital information management. The need for clinical leadership. *Br Med J* 1995;**311**:175–80.

16 The Audit Commission. *For Your Information: a study of information management in the acute hospital*. London: HMSO, 1995.

17 Lock C. What value do computers provide to the NHS hospitals. *Br Med J* 1996;**312**:1407–10.

18 Hvidt EP *et al.* Picture, archiving and communications workshop (PACS). Introducing and working with a fully digitalized radiographic service. *Orthopaedics* 1997;**5**:431–5.

19 Furedi F. *Culture of Fear: risk taking and the morality of low expectation*. London: Cassell, 1997.

20 Leape L. Cited in *Br Med J* 1997;**315**:970.

21 National Audit Office. *Health and Safety in NHS Acute Hospital Trusts in England*. London: HMSO, 1996.

22 Ennis M, Vincent CA. Obstetric accidents; a review of 64 cases. *Br Med J* 1990;**300**:1365.

23 Vincent C, Clements. Clinical risk management—why do we need it? *Clinical Risk* 1995;**1**:1–4.

24 Hiatt HH, Barnes BA, Brennan I *et al.* The study of medical injury and medical malpractice; an overview. *New Engl J Med* 1989;**321**:40.

25 Wilson RM, Runciman WB *et al.* The quality in Australian Health Care Study. *Med J Aust* 1995;**163**:458–71.

26 Editorial. *JAMA* 1998;**279**:1200.

27 NHS Confederation Action Points No. 3 October, 1997.

28 Weed LL. New connections between medical knowledge and patient care. *Br Med J* 1997;**315**:231–5.

29 National Audit Office. *Clinical Audit in England*. London: HMSO, 1995.

30 Pollock A, Evans M. *Surgical Audit*. London: Butterworth, 1989.

31 Farrell L. Audit my shorts. *Br Med J* 1995;**311**:1171.

32 Editorial. *J R Coll Physicians* 1996;**30**:415–25.

33 Berger A. Why doesn't audit work? *Br Med J* 1998;**316**:875–6.

34 Lord J, Littlejohns P. Evaluating healthcare policies: the case of clinical audit. *Br Med J* 1997;**315**:668–72.

35 Fletcher DR. Laparoscopic cholecystectomy: what national benefits have been achieved and at what cost? *Med J Aust* 1995;**163**:535–8.

36 Johnson A. Laparoscopic surgery. *Lancet* 1997;**349**:631–5.

37 Womack C, Roger S, Lavin M. Disclosure of clinical audit records in law: risk and possible defences. *Br Med J* 1996;**315**:1369–70.

38 Rangachari J. Evidence based medicine: old French wine with a new Canadian label. *J R Soc Med* 1997;**90**:280–4.

39 Sackett DL. *Br Med J* 1996;**312**:71–2.

40 Appleby J, Walshe K, Ham C. *Acting on Evidence*. NAHAT Research Paper 17, 1996.
41 *Effective Health Care*, 1996;**2**(8).
42 Muir Gray JA. Evidence based, locally owned, patient centred guideline development. *Br J Surg* 1997;**84**:1636–7.
43 Grimshaw JM, Russell IT. Effect of clinical guidelines on medical practice. *Lancet* 1993;**342**:1317–22.
44 Naylor CD. Meta-analysis and the meta-epidemiology of clinical research. *Br Med J* 1997;**315**:617–19.
45 Green J, Britten N. Qualitative research and EBM. *Br Med J* 1998;**316**:1230–2.
46 Knottnerus JA, Dinant GJ. Medicine based evidence, a prerequisite for evidence based medicine. *Br Med J* 1997;**315**:1109–10.
47 Smith GD, Egger M. Meta-analysis. Unresolved issues and further developments. *Br Med J* 1998;**316**:221–5.
48 Egger M *et al.* Bias in meta-analysis detected by a simple, graphical test. *Br Med J* 1997;**315**:629–34.
49 Egger M, Smith GD, Phillips AN. Meta-analysis. Principles and procedures. *Br Med J* 1997;**315**:1533–7.
50 Le Lorier J *et al. New Engl J Med* 1997;**337**:536–42.
51 Editorial. *Lancet* 1992;**339**:1197–8.
52 Editorial. *Lancet* 1997;**350**:675.
53 Tracey JM *et al. Br Med J* 1997;**315**:1426–8.
54 Platt R. *Private and Controversial*. London: Cassell, 1972, p. 124.
55 Kerridge I *et al.* Ethics and evidence based medicine. *Br Med J* 1998;**316**:1151.
56 Sackett DL. EBM what it is and what it is not. *Br Med J* 1996;**312**:71–2.
57 Mann T. *Clinical Guidelines*. NHS Executive, May 1996.
58 *Bolitho v City and Hackney Health Authority. The Times Law Report* 27 November 1997.
59 Grol R. Beliefs and evidence in changing clinical practice. *Br Med J* 1997;**315**:418–21.
60 Dunning M, Lugon M, McDonald J. Is clinical effectiveness a management issue. *Br Med J* 1998;**316**:243–4.
61 Durand-Zaleski I, Colin C, Blum-Boisgard C. An attempt to save money by using mandatory practice guidelines in France. *Br Med J* 1997;**315**:943–6.
62 Fairfield *et al. Br Med J* 1997;**314**:1823–6.
63 Fairfield *et al. Br Med J* 1997;**314**:1895–8.
64 Fairfield *et al. Br Med J* 1997;**315**:50–3.
65 McArthur, Moore. The two cultures and the health care revolution. *JAMA* 1997;**277**:985–9.
66 Quoted by Fairfield. *Br Med J* 1997;**314**:1896.
67 House of Lords Select Committee on Science and Technology. *Priorities in Medical Research*. London: HMSO, 1988.
68 Department of Health. *Research for Health*. London: HMSO, 1991.
69 NHS Executive. *Strategic Framework for the Use of the NHS R&D Levy*. January 1997.

70 Last JM. Making the dictionary of epidemiology. *Int J Epidemiol* 1996; **25**:1098–101.
71 Culyer A. *Supporting Research and Development in the NHS*. London: HMSO, 1994.
72 Department of Health. *Department of Health and NHS Funding for Research and Development*. London: HMSO, 1997.
73 Department of Health. *A First Class Service: quality in the new NHS*. London: HMSO, 1998.
74 Porter R. *The Greatest Benefit to Mankind: a medical history of humanity*. London: Harper Collins, 1997.
75 *The Daily Telegraph* 3 July 1998.
76 Barton A. Conditional fees: access to justice for all. *Clinical Risk* 1997; **3**:130–1.
77 Jones MA. *Medical Negligence*, 2nd edn. London: Sweet and Maxwell, 1996.
78 Baird RN. The vascular patient as litigant. *Ann R Coll Surg Engl* 1996; **78**(suppl):278–87.
79 Lord Woolf. *Access to Justice*. London: HMSO, 1996.
80 Lord Woolf. Changing landscapes in medical negligence. *Clinical Risk* 1997;**3**:202–4.
81 Lord Otton. A three-stage scheme for medical negligence. *J R Soc Med* 1998;**91**:421–6.

Worthwhile reading

Baker MR, Kirk S. *Research and Development for the NHS*, 2nd edn. Oxford: Radcliffe Medical Press, 1998.
Muir Gray JA. *Evidence Based Healthcare*. New York: Churchill Livingstone, 1997.

7 The Future

7.1 The future of medical management

Predicting the future is a dangerous business because most predictions end up wrong, but in the matter of the future world of the medical manager I think we can see a fair way ahead. Indeed if they are about to take off flight crews ought to be able to see to the end of the runway at least.

7.1.1 Medical management will survive

It is reasonable to ask whether clinicians will continue to be involved in management in the future. It is prudent to ask why they might not wish to continue. One reason for withdrawal would be as a consequence of the general change in the attitude of doctors to service. There are many factors altering the relationship of doctors with their job and with their patients, of which the interference of the state is only one. Changes in hours, lack of continuity, defensiveness formalised in risk management and a general lack of societal feeling all contribute. Doctors have always committed a lot to medicine and for most it is the all engaging passion of their lives and that is one of the things that leads them into the peripheral commitments of research, publishing, committee work and, more recently, management. Calman programmes will one presumes deliver future consultants who are younger and more narrowly trained into posts which are more specialist and more driven by protocol and dictat than is the case now. Such doctors will need the stimulus of variability in their careers and time in a managerial post will surely form one of the options for "career development" for these people. By contrast, if the combination of general social change and a continuing interposition of non-clinical agencies between doctors and their work continues, they may increasingly become less vocational, more a nine to fiver, and less willing to take on extra work. One is already noting some difficulties in recruiting doctors into management posts as the first wave step down. In my experience the reasons for this are many, but they boil down to the hassles, the conflict of loyalties and, lastly, an unwillingness for most of them to become involved in those parts of management which are not really related to patient care. Of course they could always be bribed back by the right payment but that would be the wrong reason for their involvement. This is a gloomy scenario and my preferred prediction is that their natural streaks of leadership and curiosity will continue to ensure the recruitment of doctors into management.

7.1.2 The medical manager of the future

The roles of medical managers as currently practised have in general evolved rather than been specified centrally or developed on the basis of historical experience. We can expect that role to evolve in the future as experience grows and clinicians who have "gone into management" build on their experience better to define the roles of their successors. The majority of those successors will need to be not just clinicians co-opted to be managers to give credibility and support to the management process, but will need to be separate animals. As such I suggest that most will not want to spend their time worrying about the details of finance and personnel, the negotiating of contracts and marketing and the monitoring of compliance. They will want their involvement to be primarily, perhaps even exclusively, in the areas which non-clinical managers cannot so easily understand: quality and performance, education, and the strategy for delineating optimal care and the needs of patients. *Doctors should do what only doctors can do.*

So there will be clinicians in management. What may then preoccupy them? Let me guess at the following:

(1) *Everything thus far described in this book.* I doubt if any of the difficulties to do with making teams work, adapting to limited resources, improving quality and performance will disappear.
(2) *Accountability* and a changed view of *professionalism.*
(3) *Scientism versus humanism.*
(4) *Education.*
(5) *The shape and style of the NHS.*

There are of course other things that will preoccupy them as doctors. The growth of team working, the march of technology, the tide of information and how to handle it, the shift into primary care if there is to be one, or perhaps the shift back from primary care into secondary care. Who knows, but these are general concerns of doctors and this book is about medical management.

7.2 Accountability

It is said that we are now in the third health revolution. The first was the arrival of technology to improve care, the second the impact of financial constraints, the third the era of accountability.[1] The pressure for accountability could in the future see medical care going in one of two directions, either deprofessionalised, over-regulated, over-audited, a further slip into a morass of bureaucracy, or it could adopt a new respect for redefined professionalism where doctors, nurses and others are trusted to deliver the best care they can in the circumstances, the whole process being constructively monitored and reviewed as distinct from policed. Doctors in management, if they remain primarily doctors and keep their nerve, will be well positioned to catalyse these latter changes. Politicians, purchasers and the public, as well as other professionals, will need to accept that professionalism is something to be cherished, not subverted. Doctors, like other professionals, will need to maintain their pride in being professionals, keep a positive grip on it. To quote Peter Hennessy:[2]

> for years I have nurtured a speculation that future scholars might see in eighties and nineties Britain a malign factor at work—loss of nerve about those activities and institutions in which we could still claim to be truly worldclass. ... The crumbling of our self-confidence as a professional society has led to breaches appearing in our institutional walls through which has marched an assertive army, management consultants, accountants and self-proclaimed reformers who evangelically recite the latest acronymic babble ... My embryonic thesis about institutional nerve loss ... depicts its beneficiaries as "The Three Horsemen of the Contemporary Apocalypse; Money, Management and Marketing". All three, as they ride in brandishing their crude performance indicators, are quite incapable of appreciating that ... the whole is greater than the sum of the parts; that's the point of institutions—we do

together what we cannot do alone. The eighties and nineties have seen the thoughts of those who actually do the work written off as "producer views" which must be discounted, as they are driven by vested interest. And, sadly, there were enough genuine inefficiencies and restrictive practices to give the managerialists a case. But all too often you had the sense that the reformers disliked, even despised, the objects of their zeal—thinking that, at best, they needed saving from themselves and, at worse, they required punishing for past under-performance.

That was not written about medicine and the Health Service but it applies to that institution as closely as it does to those to which it referred.

These threats are not temporary ones. They leave with us a legacy of a third force in our institutions, an increasingly powerful group of people who do not carry out any of the core functions but merely monitor, analyse, hypothesise and direct. They have too vested a personal interest to be easily displaced and like so many computer viruses become an integral if unhelpful part of the operations of the machine. A new generation of doctors may come to regard them as a natural feature of a landscape and be untroubled. But to be thus untroubled they will need to know them and their ways well and cooperate or confound them as is appropriate. This sounds like an echo of the antimanagerialism deprecated in Chapter 1 of this book, but it is not. It is a desire to keep as much of the decision making in healthcare as close to those who carry out the work as possible, and that means those who have daily contact with patients, i.e. clinicians, nurses and other professionals, for I believe only these people can truly concentrate on what the patients need and want. Nevertheless, if doctors are going to go on claiming that right of primacy then they will need to polish up their act as far as patients are concerned. *Clean* up their act you might say and this means not taking the relationship with patients too much for granted. It means working harder to prove that they can be trusted to do the best for the patient. The list of issues arising from the Bristol case identified by the General Medical Council (GMC) (Table 7.1) is a good checklist for any doctor or manager wishing to approach this issue formally.

The NHS at present has the huge virtue that it allows patients to believe that doctors and others within it are not doing things to them or for them simply for financial gain. Nevertheless if we

274

Table 7.1 Issues of clinical governance raised by the Bristol Cardiothoracic Surgery case and identified by the GMC

- The need for clearly understood clinical standards
- How clinical competence and technical expertise are assessed and evaluated
- Who carries the responsibility in team-based care
- The training of doctors in advanced procedures
- How to approach the so-called learning curve of doctors undertaking established procedures
- The reliability and validity of the data used to monitor doctors' personal performance
- The use of medical and clinical audit
- The appreciation of the importance of factors, other than purely clinical ones, that can affect clinical judgment, performance and outcome
- The responsibility of a consultant to take appropriate actions in response to concerns about his or her performance
- The factors which appear to discourage openness and frankness about doctors' personal performance
- How doctors explain risks to patients
- The ways in which people concerned about patient safety can make their concerns known
- The need for doctors to take prompt action at an early stage where a colleague is in difficulty, in order to offer the best chance of avoiding damage to patients and the colleague, and of putting things right

---

(Reproduced from *GMC News* 1998;**3**)

consider the darker sides of the Patient's Charter, the culture of complaint and the rise of selfish and individualistic consumerism, the doctor–patient relationship can become positively adversarial. Medical managers can do as much as anyone to keep the relationship on the rails. At present it sometimes seems that the expected way that doctor–patient relationships will be improved is through formal education of staff. There is a great danger that in pursuing that the educational theorists advising the GMC and the medical schools will over-egg the curriculum insisting on early and formal training in ethics, social and legal issues. I am not convinced that the full monty legal and ethical curriculum proposed by a consensus group of clinicians, philosophers, lawyers and theologians and put out as "non-negotiable"[3] will really do what is needed. The authors have presumably not seen how easy it is to "turn off" undergraduates and trainees by heavy-handed formal education in these topics. By contrast the medical manager, together with undergraduate and postgraduate tutors, can make sure that these topics are drip-fed into all trainees through the medium of communications, seminars, audit meetings, and committee agendas throughout training so the issues are seen in context.

In establishing accountability and redefining professionalism part of the deal which the professional will need to make with the public goes beyond tightening up professional competence and self regulation. It involves (and this is the bit the management books forget to mention) somehow reassuring patients that doctors are still on their side while not concealing the constraints. Doctors who have been medical mangers will, one hopes, desist from the unfortunate habit that many non-managerial clinicians have, of negatively emphasising to the patients the resource problems, saying how awful the Department of Health, the purchasers and the managers are. The mature clinician will need to explain the difficulties while making it clear to the patient that he remains on his side. In this the doctor's role is no different from when he is treating diseases. When faced with a patient with a new diagnosis of cancer of the bronchus, one hopes most clinicians do not launch into a denigration of the fickleness of God, the venality of tobacco manufacturers, the shocking lack of a screening programme, and the slowness of the referring GP. The clinician focuses on what can be achieved for the patient.

7.3 Scientism versus humanism

This was ever a problem for doctors. Technology, the military arm of science, always carries risk to patients as well as benefits, particularly when it articulates the habit of action in preference to reflection. Evidence-based medicine (EBM), managed care and protocols will be culturally dominant in the lives of doctors soon, extending the tentacles of scientific truism further into the soft corners of medical art. In our fixation on its benefits we may lose the subtleties that distinguish the profession of medicine from the profession of engineering or of physics. It is not just that we may lose humanity but we may also lose some subtlety of perception—"the concept is always the enemy of intuition".[4] By identifying the disease and by automatically translating it into a protocol, we potentially lose our ability to see the patient, just as when we call a thrush a thrush, or a willow a willow, we may cease to see the bird or the tree for its true self.

But enough of this namby-pamby stuff!

The hard area of EBM will be its imposition or otherwise in day-to-day care. Swales, in his essay on "Culture and medicine"[5] has stressed the importance of realising that health involves more than "scientism" (i.e. the belief that science-based evidence can resolve all the difficulties of the health service). He reminds us that we cannot extrapolate scientific absolutism to the relativism of cultural values, that society is heterogeneous, that individuals have different assessments of what they want and what they will tolerate. In her role as the go between, between managerialism and the patient, the medical manager will need to develop her role as the arbiter in the imposition of an increasingly structured set of rules about what should be done to whom, when and at what cost. She may be the focal point of debate about care which bounces back and forth between what *can* be done, what the protocol says *should* be done and what *ought* to be done for this particular patient. Establishing herself as the person within the organisation who has the right to make those judgments may be more difficult. As go between she will also need to grapple with a shift from a service led (you get what we provide) to a needs led (you get what you say you want) service, which is the consumerist face of a more patient-orientated service. One of the great stimuli to team working should be that it will refine these professionally human judgments and also give them more clout.

7.4 Education

Education you may say is not the business of the medical manager but if he is to intercede between the patient-focused world of clinicians and the resource-focused world of managers, he will need to educate both parties, not in a sense of formal lectures but the continuing education of giving facts, putting views and changing attitudes and behaviour. In her paper on changes in continuing medical education, Angela Towle summarised the responsiveness needed of medical education as follows:

- Teach scientific behaviour as well as scientific facts.
- Promote the use of information technology.
- Adapt to the change in doctor–patient relationship.
- Help future doctors to shape and adapt to change.
- Promote multiprofessional team working and care.
- Help future doctors handle broader responsibilities.
- Reflect the changing pattern of disease and healthcare delivery.
- Involve health service employers and users.

277

It is difficult to envisage a situation where the medical manager is not a prime participant in that sort of educational process.[6]

7.5 The shape and style of the NHS

The hospital as an institution has come to dominate the NHS; since its inception their share of the budget rising from 54% in 1948 to 70% by the mid 1970s. The main thrust of the trend to involve doctors in management has come within hospitals, which one might think lend themselves to being manageable units easily managed. However it has, as this book has intimated, been very difficult and is only just achieving a fragile existence as a working system. Yet the trends suggest that the future of the NHS lies in deconstructing its current arrangements and developing new ones where teams link up across traditional boundaries to provide a host of integrated care networks. It all sounds persuasive and worthy, but little is written about how such systems might be managed in a day-to-day way and by whom. If this is to be the shape of the future Health Service we will need to define how primary care and hospitals will manage the processes that can deliver seamlessly managed patterns of care.

A new government was elected in 1997 and the phraseology of documents about the Health Service changed. There was less talk of competition and cost and marketing. New headlines were about cooperation and equity and the White Paper of December 1997, "The New NHS: Modern and Dependable" seemed to be heading in the right direction but with a new flush of quangos, promises of more money and, running through it, still the old controlling reflex, mixed with the socialist instinct to make everything the same. These instincts have some benefits for all that. The prospect of more sensible planning for specialist services and of longer-term budgeting and service agreements bodes well and implies that management within the Health Service may in a practical sense be easier if the pace of change is manageable. The White Paper planned the removal of a billion pounds from the administrative side of healthcare but does not outline explicitly how this will be achieved, nor do other provisions within the White Paper leave any leeway for reducing management costs. The performance and quality management initiatives will require substantial clinical and non-clinical managerial input. Whether the implication is that more managerial functions will be devolved onto professionals within the service is again unclear.

We are told that what the public wants is convenience, quality and explicitness. If the government will fund it and the medical profession engage properly in the management of its delivery, then there is no reason why the public should not get what it wants and have it provided by a re-energised medical profession.

References

1 Relman AS. Assessment and accountability. *New Engl J Med* 1988;**319**: 1220–2.
2 Hennessy P. Book review of "Utopia and Other Places" by Sir Richard Eyre. *The Independent* 22 January 1997.
3 Doyal N, Gillon R. Medical ethics and law as a core subject in medical education. *Br Med J* 1998;**316**:1623–4.
4 Roose-Evans J. *Inner Journey, Outer Journey*. London: Darton, Longman, Todd, 1998, p. 185.
5 Swales J. Culture and medicine. *J R Soc Med* 1998;**91**:118–26.
6 Towle A. Changes in healthcare and continuing medical education for the 21st century. *Br Med J* 1998;**316**:301–4.

Index